# ROLE OF POTASSIUM IN PREVENTIVE CARDIOVASCULAR MEDICINE

# BASIC SCIENCE FOR THE CARDIOLOGIST

1.  B. Swynghedauw (ed.): *Molecular Cardiology for the Cardiologist*. Second Edition. 1998.                           ISBN: 0-7923-8323-0

2.  B. Levy, A. Tedgui (eds.): *Biology of the Arterial Wall*. 1999
                                               ISBN 0-7923-8458-X

3.  M.R. Sanders, J.B. Kostis (eds): *Molecular Cardiology in Clinical Practice*. 1999.                           ISBN 0-7923-8602-7

4.  B. Ostadal, F. Kolar (eds.): *Cardiac Ischemia: From Injury to Protection*. 1999
                                               ISBN 0-7923-8642-6

5.  H. Schunkert, G.A.J. Riegger (eds.): *Apoptosis in Cardiac Biology*. 1999.
                                               ISBN 0-7923-8648-5
6.  A. Malliani, (ed.): *Principles of Cardiovascular Neural Regulation in Health and Disease*.                           ISBN 0-7923-7775-3

7.  P. Benlian : G*enetics of Dyslipidemia*. 2001

                                               ISBN 0-7923-7362-6

8.  D. Young : *Role of Potassium in Preventive Cardiovascular Medicine*. 2001
                                               ISBN 0-7923-7376-6

KLUWER ACADEMIC PUBLISHERS - DORDRECHT/BOSTON/LONDON

# ROLE OF POTASSIUM IN PREVENTIVE CARDIOVASCULAR MEDICINE

*by*

**David B. Young, Ph.D.**
*University of Mississippi Medical Center, U.S.A.*

**KLUWER ACADEMIC PUBLISHERS**
**Boston / Dordrecht / London**

**Distributors for North, Central and South America:**
Kluwer Academic Publishers
101 Philip Drive
Assinippi Park
Norwell, Massachusetts 02061 USA

**Distributors for all other countries:**
Kluwer Academic Publishers Group
Distribution Centre
Post Office Box 322
3300 AH Dordrecht, THE NETHERLANDS

**Library of Congress Cataloging-in-Publication Data**

Young, David B.
    Role of potassium in preventive cardiovascular medicine / by David B. Young.
      p. ; cm. – (Basic Science for the cardiologist ; 8)
    Includes bibliographical references and index.
    ISBN 0-7923-7376-6 (alk. paper)
      1.   Cardiovascular system--Pathophysiology. 2. Cardiovascular
system--Diseases--Prevention. 3. Potassium--Physiological effect. I. Title. II. Series.
    [DNLM: 1. Cardiovascular Diseases--prevention & control. 2. Cardiovascular
Physiology. 3.Potassium--physiology.4. Potassium--therapeutic use. WG 120 Y69r 2001]
    RC669.9 . Y68 2001
    616.1'05--dc21                              200135419

*Printed on acid-free paper.*

Printed in the United States of America

*The Publisher offers discounts on this book for bulk purchases. For further
information, send email to [laura.walsh@wkap.com]*

For

Susan,

Brian, Matthew and Sara

# CONTENTS

## SECTION II:    CARDIOVASCULAR RESPONSES TO CHANGES IN POTASSIUM

*page ix*

# FOREWORD

To me, ionic potassium existing in body fluids comprises one of the most interesting substances in biology. Potassium is also one of the most abundant substances present in all plant and animal life. There are about 3,500 mmol of potassium in the body. But, just as in plant life, most of these potassium ions reside inside the cell wherein their osmotic action helps sustain cell volume. There are about equal amounts of sodium ions in the body, which in contrast, largely reside outside the cells where by osmotic and hydraulic action they sustain the volume or amount of fluid present in the blood plasma, and via the Dohnan equilibrium, also the amount of fluid in the extracellular spaces baiting the tissues.

But the similarities stop there. Apart from its essential osmotic role, sodium is apparently largely inert biologically, although there are those who believe that besides its osmotic hydraulic actions, a sodium volume excess can somehow induce or sustained arteriolar vasoconstriction and thereby sustain high blood pressure.

Potassium is quite another story. The small amounts of potassium, only 65 mmol, that exist in the blood and extracellular fluids are extremely active electrophysiologically and metabolically, so that very small acute changes in the plasma potassium level can have profound effects, rapidly producing changes in cardiac rhythm and even cardiac arrest, an effect exploited by cardiac surgeons to perform open heart surgery.

Potassium also plays a major role in nerve conduction and for enabling skeletal and cardiac muscle contraction. Because of all these properties, wise clinicians have long avoided giving rapid intravenous infusions of potassium.

Nature protects us from the dangerous effects of rapidly ingested potassium by providing an energy requiring transport system, involving sodium, potassium-ATPase that continuously pumps sodium out of the cell allowing potassium to enter in its place. Besides this fundamental transport system, nature has evolved an elaborate hormonal control system, the renin-angiotensin-aldosterone system, which closely defends plasma potassium concentration together with body sodium balance and the arterial blood pressure level. Thus, when you or I eat a large potassium meal, e.g.: a large beef steak or a large glass of orange juice, when the plasma potassium concentration rises by only 0.3 mmol/L or less, this stimulates the adrenal cortical secretion of aldosterone that promptly acts on the distal tubules to promote kaliuresis, thereby restoring body potassium and plasma potassium levels back to normal. Thus, patients with Addison's Disease whose cortex cannot make enough aldosterone can develop dangerous hyperkalemia with cardiac arrest.

I hope my brief orientation will help the reader to perhaps better enjoy the valuable aggregation of historical data on the many potentially exciting roles of potassium intake on major hypertensive and cardiovascular disorders. Dr. Young's thoughtful compendium on this information is also spiced by timely presentations of his own creative research on the roles of potassium in cardiovascular function. We're only beginning to understand potassium and its roles in human biology, and in particular in human hypertensive cardiovascular and diabetic disorders. Having David Young's book at your side will make the potassium story more understandable and more exciting for the curious biologist or physician.

I have followed David Young's research with admiration for some 25 years. We've known each other since the days when my research group used to visit Arthur Guyton, David's mentor. We met for two or three days in Jackson and discussed eachother's experiments. We had many great exchanges during which David's perspicacity and future research potentials were already apparent.

Accordingly, David's book is a must for me and all other Kalomaniacs.

John H. Laragh, M.D.
Director, Cardiovascular Center
New York Presbyterian Hospital-
Weill Medical College of Cornell University

# Chapter 1

# INTRODUCTION

Coronary artery disease, stroke, and other forms of cardiovascular pathology are the leading causes of death in industrialized nations, accounting for approximately half of all mortality. Through myocardial ischemia, heart failure and cerebral infarction, cardiovascular diseases cripple, weaken and otherwise rob the quality from the lives of tens of millions, sometimes for decades before the final morbid aspect of the disease. Accordingly, research directed to finding causes, preventative measures and cures for these diseases has received high priority in the countries of the industrialized world.

Prevention of disease is always better than a cure; however, the largest share of our health care expenditure is devoted to curative rather than preventative measures. For cardiovascular disease, the greatest benefit to the population thus far has come from treatments, such as coronary artery bypass surgery, coronary artery angioplasty, and antihypertensive medications. Testing and designing approaches to prevent cardiovascular disease have been difficult for several reasons, including that the studies required to establish effectiveness may take years to complete, and rarely provide unequivocal answers. However, almost daily we encounter claims for preventative effectiveness attributable to products ranging from vegetables to vitamins, generally in the absence of adequate scientific analytical support but in the presence of ample presumptive, media hype.

The public has given relatively little attention to the potential importance of potassium as a protective component of the diet. However, for several decades, evidence has accumulated from analytical studies suggesting that high levels of dietary potassium intake may be protective against development of cardiovascular diseases.  While no single study has produced the exciting elucidation of truth that attracts media attention, the sum of the scientific reports has become more and more convincing.

The significance of potassium depletion in cardiovascular disease in modern man may be best appreciated in light of our ancestry.  The human genome was selected in an environment that provided our progenitors with a diet containing high levels of potassium and low levels of sodium, compared to the modern diet.  Associated with this limited supply of sodium was the development of a highly effective sodium appetite, and a powerful system for conserving sodium once it was ingested.  But unlike the developed responses to the sodium-poor environment, no effective systems evolved for potassium appetite or conservation.  Consequently, the members of modern industrialized cultures select diets rich in sodium and poor in potassium, and live in a state of relative potassium depletion most of their lives.

A diet similar to that of our prehistoric ancestors is consumed today by primitive populations that persist in hunter-gather cultures.  These groups eat unrefined foods providing intake rates from 20 to 40 mmol/day for sodium and 200-300 mmol/day for potassium, whereas the daily intake of potassium and sodium for individuals of industrialized cultures eating processed foods is 80 to 250 mmol/day for sodium and 20 to 70 mmol/day for potassium.  The diets and epidemiology of at least 14 of these primitive cultures from all corners of the globe have been studied in detail.  In none is the incidence of hypertension greater than 1%, coronary artery disease and congestive heart failure are nearly unknown, and strokes are rare occurrences.  These groups, which are from several continents, and which include genetic diversity overlapping the gene pool of industrialized societies, have nearly complete protection from the cardiovascular diseases that account for one-half of the deaths in developed cultures.

Numerous differences exist between the diets of primitive groups and of industrial societies besides the potassium and sodium content, any or all of which may contribute to the protection against cardiovascular disease.  The primitive, unrefined diet has a lower fat content, lower caloric density, lower levels of trace elements and food processing additives, and higher amounts of fiber. The importance of any one of these as a causative factor contributing to the differences in cardiovascular disease rates has not been established. However, evidence supporting a protective role for high potassium intake has been reported persistently during the last 90 years. Consistent with the hypothesis are findings from a variety of disciplines including anthropology, epidemiology, clinical intervention trials, population-based research and animal experimentation. And in the last few years, results from analyses of the impact of physiologic changes in potassium concentration on the cells of cardiovascular tissues have added to the understanding of the basic mechanisms that may be affected by potassium to account for its cardiovascular protective actions.

At this point, the available information compels us to consider seriously the question of whether an elevation of potassium intake can be protective against cardiovascular disease in individuals and in populations, and if so, should recommendation be made that potassium intake be increased in patients at risk and/or in the general population. To give due consideration to these questions requires integration of findings from many fields gained through several decades of study. Because of the complex nature of the information that should be considered, and because of the potential importance of the answers to the questions raised, I consider it appropriate to present the most pertinent background as a monograph directed to leaders of the cardiovascular medical community, the leaders who will make the decisions concerning application of the findings. My purpose is to encourage consideration of these questions, and to stimulate posing of new ones that will lead to the definitive studies.

Material presented in the following chapters is limited to what may be useful in determining the significance of potassium in preventive cardiovascular medicine. Each chapter presents selected information concerning a topic that could be the subject of a major review article. But this monograph is not intended to be a series of the exhaustive reviews; in most chapters, references to articles providing more complete coverage are provided for the reader's convenience. Instead, my design was to bring together only the most important evidence from a broad range of disciplines that should be considered before attempting to understand the potential importance of potassium. Nor was my intention to prescribe specific medical advice for treatment of patients; I am not a physician, and therefore the reader should not infer that I recommend measures for treatment of patients.

The book is divided into two sections, the first focused upon regulation of potassium, the second dealing with specific influences of potassium on the cardiovascular system. The ability of the body to regulate potassium in responses to changes in intake is complex in that the effectiveness of control is greater at high levels of intake than at low levels, and it is affected by sodium intake. In addition, the potassium control system interacts with renal mechanisms that control sodium balance and blood pressure, and consequently, the operation of the system has the potential to affect blood pressure regulation. Furthermore, the majority of medications commonly used for treatment of cardiovascular diseases affects potassium regulation. Section I considers these topics, regulation of potassium (Chapter 2) and interactions between potassium regulation and commonly used medications (Chapter 3), and concludes with consideration of hypokalemia, its causes and remedies (Chapter 4). Section II begins with a description of responses of cells of the cardiovascular system to changes in potassium concentration (Chapter 5), information from *in vitro* studies that permitted analysis of direct effects of potassium concentration on functions of the cells. The next three chapters provide evidence from laboratory experiments, clinical studies, and population based analyses suggesting that elevation of potassium intake inhibits thrombosis and stroke (Chapter 6), arteriosclerosis and atherosclerotic lesion formation (Chapter 7), and neointimal proliferation following angioplastic balloon injury (Chapter 8). Chapter 9 considers a large body of evidence concerning the relationship between dietary potassium intake and blood pressure. Chapter 10 reviews the relationship between hypokalemia and incidence of serious ventricular arrhythmias. The impact of potassium depletion on diastolic function is presented in Chapter 11, including data from laboratory animal studies, and cardiac function studies in human volunteers. In Chapter 12, a general summary is presented, and recommendations and conclusions are proposed.

The most accurate assessment of potassium's potential can be made by incorporating the disparate findings from the many fields into a unified understanding, and therefore, I urge the reader to consider each of the chapters.

# SECTION I

# POTASSIUM REGULATION

# Chapter 2

# PHYSIOLOGY OF POTASSIUM REGULATION

## POTASSIUM TRANSPORT ALONG THE NEPHRON

## REGULATION OF POTASSIUM DISTRIBUTION

## HORMONAL AND NON-HORMONAL FACTORS THAT MAY AFFECT POTASSIUM EXCRETION AND DISTRIBUTION

## LONG-TERM REGULATION OF POTASSIUM: IMPORTANCE OF ALDOSTERONE AND EXTRACELLULAR POTASSIUM CONCENTRATION

## SYSTEMS ANALYSES OF POTASSIUM REGULATION

## SUMMARY

# POTASSIUM TRANSPORT ALONG THE NEPHRON

All life forms require a well controlled extracellular potassium concentration for normal function. In mammals the concentration in the extracellular fluid (ECF) is held in a well regulated range that deviates no more than 15% from the desired level, 4.2 mmol/L in man and most other mammals. Until relatively recently, the human diet contained several times more potassium and less sodium than the modern diet; primitive human diets contain approximately 400 mmol/day of potassium, an amount equal to approximately five times the amount present in the total ECF, and only a few mmol/day of sodium (1,2). Modern, Western diets contain 50 to 80 mmol/day of potassium, and usually 50 to 200 mmol/day of sodium (3-5). While eating either diet, ECF potassium concentration can be held within the desired, normal range during the course of each day while widely varying amounts of potassium are absorbed from the gastrointestinal tract, and over periods of many days while the rate of intake of potassium and sodium may vary from zero to extremely high rates. However, because the regulatory system evolved under conditions in which potassium intake was much higher than it is in modern diets, our ability to excrete large amounts of potassium from a potassium-rich diet is much more robust than our ability to conserve potassium from excretion when consuming a potassium-deplete diet. And consequently, while our ability to control extracellular potassium concentration is extremely competent when consuming a potassium-rich diet, our ability to control potassium concentration is relatively poor when our diet is low in potassium.

In order to control the concentration of a substance in the ECF, a system may regulate intake and excretion from the body, and the distribution within the body between the intra- and extracellular compartments. But unlike the sodium control system, the potassium system does not include regulation of intake by an appetitive mechanism, nor are absorption from and excretion into the gut subject to quantitatively important active regulation. Therefore, long-term regulation of potassium is mediated solely by controlling the rate of renal excretion, which can vary from less than 10 mmol/day to well over 400 mmol/day. Changes in distribution of potassium between the intra-and extracellular spaces can act as only a short-term buffer to perturbations in ECF concentration. Renal excretion is modulated by inherent alterations in nephron function in response to changes in plasma potassium concentration and other factors, and by changes in the concentration of hormones reaching the kidney in the blood.

## Potassium is Freely Filtered Across the Glomerular Membrane

However, the amount entering the nephron from the glomerulus has little influence on the rate of potassium excretion. Approximately 80 percent of the filtered potassium is reabsorbed in the proximal convoluted tubule along the thick ascending limb of Henle's loop. Further potassium reabsorption can take place along the distal tubule and collecting ducts when potassium conservation is required. However, under normal conditions potassium secretion occurs across the epithelium of the distal nephron and collecting ducts, especially in the most distal sections of the distal tubule (cortical connecting tubule) and the cortical portion of the collecting tubule. Cells in these tubular segments, the principal cells and the intercalated cells, respond to physiological signals by changing their rates of potassium secretion over a wide range. The principal cells secrete potassium and the intercalated cells are responsible for potassium reabsorption from the lumen. The potassium absorptive mechanisms are of limited quantitative importance in man, as evidenced by the poor capability to resist potassium depletion during extended periods of low potassium intake. Furthermore, the mechanisms of potassium reabsorption are poorly understood and have not been completely described at this time. On the other hand, the potassium secretory functions of the principal cells are extremely powerful and have been well characterized.

## The Basolateral Membrane of the Principal Cells Has a Rich Supply of Sodium, Potassium-ATPase, and a Conductive Pathway for Potassium

The enzyme system is responsible for uptake of potassium from, and extrusion of sodium into, the peritubular fluid. The enzyme operates in an electrogenic mode and responds to changes in extracellular potassium concentration, changes in extracellular pH, and variations in mineralocorticoid hormone concentration (6-9). In response to increases in aldosterone concentration, activation of the electrogenic sodium-potassium exchange results in hyperpolarization of these cells. The conductive pathway for potassium in the principal cell's basolateral membrane generates a diffusion potential for potassium ions from cell to peritubular space. The pathway plays a role in the increased rate of potassium secretion in response to stimulation by mineralocorticoid hormones. With mineralocorticoid treatment, the potassium conductance of the basolateral membrane increases. When the membrane is hyperpolarized as a result of the effect of the hormone on the sodium, potassium-ATPase, the electrogenic stimulation of the pump raises the membrane potential above the potassium equilibrium value, causing potassium ions to be driven from the peritubular fluid into the cell. This is in contrast to the situation when the pump is unstimulated and the membrane potential is below the potassium equilibrium value.

## Potassium Enters the Tubule Lumen Across the Apical Membrane, Driven by a Favorable Electrochemical Potential Gradient

Potassium-selective channels provide a route for potassium secretion from cell to lumen. Increasing the potassium concentration difference between cellular fluid and lumen, either by lowering tubular potassium concentration or by increasing cytoplasmic potassium activity, increases the rate of secretion. Increases in the rate of flow of tubular fluid through the potassium secreting portions of the distal nephron significantly increases potassium entry from the principal cells by reducing the tubular potassium concentration and increasing the diffusion gradient for potassium. This relationship between tubular flow rate and potassium excretion accounts in part for the kaliuretic effect of diuretics that act at sites proximal to the potassium secreting portions of the nephron (e.g. loop diuretics, thiazides), and for the potential kaliuretic effects of high rates of sodium intake.

The permeability of the luminal membrane for potassium is subject to regulation and plays an important part in the overall control of the rate of secretion. Permeability is increased by mineralocorticoid administration and is reduced by acidification of the lumen (7,10). Exposure to a high-potassium diet increases apical potassium conductance, whereas a diet low in potassium reduces luminal conductance. Analysis of the behavior of single potassium channels in apical membranes of isolated rabbit cortical and collecting tubules has demonstrated that the potassium channels are stimulated by elevation of intracellular calcium concentration, and that they are voltage-sensitive (11,12). Luminal membrane depolarization results in increased opening of the potassium channels. The voltage sensitivity may explain the increase in potassium conductance of the apical membrane following mineralocorticoid stimulation; the mineralocorticoid stimulation results in a reduction in the apical membrane potential that may affect the opening of the potassium channels in that membrane.

Also present in the apical membrane is a significant sodium conductance that allows sodium ions to enter the cell down a favorable concentration gradient. Therefore, entry of sodium ions can prevent the development of a diffusion potential as potassium ions diffuse in the opposite direction into the lumen. In addition, entry of sodium ions into the cytoplasm stimulates the basolaterally located sodium, potassium-ATPase, which brings potassium ions into the cytoplasm from the extracellular fluid. Therefore, the sodium permeability of the apical cell membrane is an important component of the mechanism for secretion of potassium. Mineralocorticoid hormones increase apical sodium permeability (7,13). Amiloride, which is extremely effective in inhibiting secretion of potassium, acts by blocking apical sodium conductance.

## Extracellular Potassium Concentration is the Most Potent Regulatory Factor in Potassium Homeostasis

Extracellular potassium has potent effects on sodium, potassium-ATPase activity, especially in the potassium secreting portions of the distal nephron. These effects are not the result of mass action effects of potassium binding to the pump. Instead, increases in $[K^+]$, up to at least 7.5 mmol/L, cause increased membrane surface density of sodium, potassium-ATPase (ouabain binding) within as little as 5 minutes (14).

# REGULATION OF POTASSIUM DISTRIBUTION

A number of factors *affect* potassium distribution and excretion but are not part of the system that *controls* the ECF concentration and renal excretion of the ion. For example, insulin and epinephrine both acutely and transiently stimulate transfer of potassium from the extra- to the intracellular space. However, these hormones are not part of the control system, for changes in potassium concentration within the physiological range do not affect the rates of secretion of the hormones (for review, see references 15 and 16). Therefore, changes in the concentrations of epinephrine and insulin often represent problems for the control system and are not part of the solution. These hormones are key elements in negative feedback control systems that operate to maintain control of other variables in the body; when, for example, insulin levels are strongly elevated in the postprandial period, its effect on potassium distribution can cause a sharp fall in potassium concentration. Similarly, during periods of cardiovascular stress, such as following myocardial infarction, extremely high levels of epinephrine present in the circulation can shift potassium from the extracellular to the intracellular space and reduce plasma potassium concentration to very low levels. Clearly, these hormones are not acting to control potassium concentration, but rather are creating short-term disturbances in the regulation of potassium.

## Aldosterone has Significant Effects on Long-Term Regulation of Potassium Distribution between the Intracellular and Extracellular Compartment

Observations from a number of experimental studies indicate that aldosterone can affect potassium distribution over extended periods. For example, in a study by Pan and Young (17) five times the normal level of aldosterone was infused into dogs for 14 days. There were no measurable changes in potassium excretion or intake during the infusion period, although plasma potassium concentration fell from 4.8 to 3.2 mmol/L, a 33-percent decrease in plasma K, with no apparent change in total body K. Young and Jackson analyzed the effect of aldosterone on potassium distribution more rigorously in two additional groups of experiments (18). In the first, dogs received continuous infusion of aldosterone at five times the normal rate, 250 micrograms/day. Total exchangeable potassium (Ke) and plasma potassium concentration were measured prior to, as well as 4 and 6 days after, the beginning of aldosterone infusion. Plasma potassium concentration fell by 20 percent, whereas Ke decreased by 8 percent after 6 days of infusion; the ratio between extracellular and total body potassium had been altered by the aldosterone infusion. In the second study, 10 adrenalectomized dogs received aldosterone infusion at a rate of 50 micrograms/day, then at 250 micrograms/day. On each level of aldosterone infusion, three levels of potassium intake were given by intravenous infusions. When the animals were in electrolyte balance at each level of aldosterone and potassium intake (after at least seven days on each level of infusion), Ke and plasma potassium concentration were measured. The two variables were plotted against each other, with Ke being the independent variable. These relationships are presented in Figure 2.1.

At the normal level of exchangeable potassium (approximately 42 mmol/kg in the dog), plasma potassium concentration can be predicted to be 4.26 mmol/L when aldosterone levels are normal. However, when aldosterone levels are increased fivefold, at the same total exchangeable potassium level, predicted plasma potassium concentration would be 3.69 mmol/L.

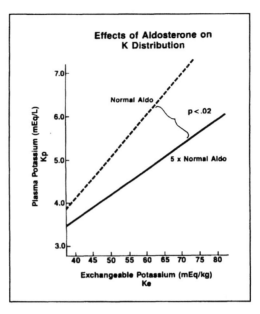

*Figure 2.1*

*Effect of aldosterone on potassium distribution. The relationship between total body potassium and plasma potassium concentration was determined in adrenalectomized dogs maintained with either normal aldosterone replacement (norm aldo), or with five times the normal level (5 x normal aldo). From reference 18.*

Data from the experiments are consistent with the hypothesis that aldosterone alters the distribution of potassium between the intra- and extracellular spaces, with a greater portion of total potassium being intracellular at higher levels of aldosterone. By this mechanism, aldosterone can alter plasma potassium concentration sufficiently to affect other components of the regulatory system, even if there is initially no change in potassium balance.

Several physiological variables are known to be capable of affecting the distribution of potassium. The hormones insulin (16,19) and epinephrine (15,20) both can induce rapid, large inward shifts of potassium, while extracellular acidosis can induce movement of potassium from the intracellular to the extracellular fluid. However, there is reason to believe that these variables are more important in affecting potassium concentration over periods of minutes and hours than during long-term control situations that pertain to the subject of this monograph. Two large patient populations provide information concerning the minimal long-term importance of epinephrine and insulin. Long-term beta adrenergic blockade appears to have only minor effects on regulation of plasma potassium concentration in hypertensive patients. Diabetic patients uncomplicated by metabolic acidosis also have apparently normal potassium control capability, and their ability to maintain regulation of potassium is unaffected by long-term changes in their insulin levels. Certainly, catecholamines and insulin are capable of affecting potassium distribution under many circumstances such as during the response to stress and during the postprandial period. But the contribution of these hormones to long-term potassium regulation remains open to question. Likewise, short-term changes in pH can affect potassium distribution, although over periods of days and weeks, pH status is well controlled and can by considered to be constant under steady-state conditions.

# HORMONAL AND NON-HORMONAL FACTORS THAT MAY AFFECT POTASSIUM EXCRETION AND DISTRIBUTION

## Sodium Intake and Excretion

Changes in sodium intake are usually not associated with large changes in potassium excretion in normal individuals. However, we observed that under some conditions elevation of sodium intake can produce a very significant increase in excretion of potassium. We analyzed this effect of sodium intake in adrenalectomized dogs that received fixed, normal rates of aldosterone replacement (normal for normal electrolyte intake, which in the 20 kg laboratory dog was 30 mmol/day of sodium and potassium) together with three levels of sodium intake, 10 to 100 and 200 mmol/day (21). While receiving the fixed level of sodium and aldosterone, potassium intake was changed from 10 to 200 mmol/day in four steps of seven to ten days duration. Plasma potassium concentration and the daily rate of potassium excretion were measured at the end of each period when the animals had achieved a state of balance. Using this design permitted analysis of the effects of changes in sodium intake and excretion on potassium excretion, without participation of changes in aldosterone concentration. Sodium intake had a striking multiplicative interaction with the kaliuretic effect of plasma potassium concentration, as presented in Figure 2.2.

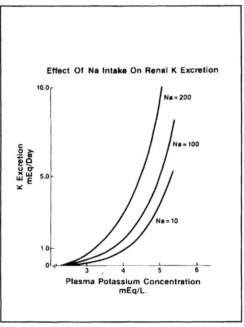

**Figure 2.2**

*The relationship between sodium intake and steady-state potassium excretion in dogs. Three levels of sodium were given, 10, 100, and 200 meq/day. From reference 21.*

Based on these data obtained when sodium intake was the only variable affecting potassium excretion that was altered, one can predict that if plasma potassium concentration were held constant at 4.0 mmol/L, increasing sodium intake from 10 to 100 mmol/day would increase steady state potassium excretion from 17 to 37 mmol/day, and further elevation of sodium intake to 200 mmol/day would raise potassium excretion to 47 mmol/day. If potassium were held constant at 4.5 mmol/L, the same increases in sodium intake would be associated with elevation of potassium excretion from 34 to 63 to 91 mmol/day.

Figure 2.3 is a three dimensional representation of the interaction between the kaliuretic effects of plasma potassium concentration and sodium intake, with normalized sodium intake and plasma potassium concentration depicted as the independent variables, and normalized potassium excretion as the dependent variable.

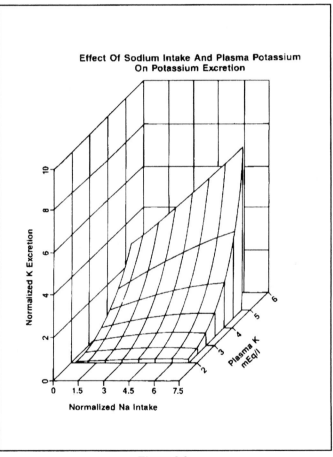

*Figure 2.3*

*Interaction between potassium concentration and sodium intake in affecting steady-state potassium excretion. Sodium intake and potassium excretion rates are normalized, with 1.0 being the normal rate. From reference 21.*

# Epinephrine

Epinephrine is associated with beta-2 agonist-induced hypokalemia and appears to protect against exercise-induced hyperkalemia (22). The effects of epinephrine may result from a combination of increased membrane potassium conductance and increased sodium, potassium-ATPase activity (23,24). Increased potassium uptake through pump activation more than offsets increased potassium efflux through the activated conductance, so that epinephrine elevates both intracellular potassium activity and the electrochemical driving force for potassium exit ($E^K$). The effects of epinephrine are primarily associated with beta-2 receptors, although beta-1 receptors agonists appear to mediate similar effects in some instances.

# Norepinephrine

In the distal convoluted tubules norepinephrine can stimulate sodium, potassium-ATPase activity through alpha-2 receptors that activate protein kinase C, rather than inhibiting adenylate cyclase (25,26). Perhaps the reported protein kinase C -mediated effect of norepinephrine on sodium, potassium-ATPase creates a sufficiently large change in the electrochemical gradient favoring sodium entry as to overcome the reported inhibition of the apical sodium channel by protein kinase C. If so, the dominance of one effect or the other on distal convoluted tubule sodium reabsorption may be critically dependent on other factors influencing sodium entry and pump activity.

# Vasopressin

Vasopressin-sensitive adenylate cyclase activity is increased by aldosterone in both the short- and long-term (27). Vasopressin itself can induce sodium absorption and potassium secretion and acts synergistically with aldosterone to increase sodium entry and sodium, potassium-ATPase activity, the latter effect being apparently secondary to increased apical sodium entry (28,29).

The mechanism of synergism is said to lie in the fact that vasopressin increases surface density of the sodium channel, whereas aldosterone increases the open probability of the same sodium channel.

## Insulin

Insulin and potassium co-vary in anephric animals, and it has been suggested that insulin and potassium interact in a feedback control system (16,30). In addition, insulin stimulates potassium secretion by the cortical collecting duct (31). Stimulation of sodium absorption by insulin can also contribute to increased potassium secretion for reasons discussed earlier. In isolated epithelial monolayers of cultured A6 and TB6C cells, insulin and aldosterone have additive effects to stimulate sodium absorption (32), and insulin stimulates sodium absorption in the medullary thick ascending limb through apparent activation of a cyclic AMP-dependent protein kinase.

An effect of insulin on regulation of plasma potassium concentration or long-term potassium balance has not been documented. In some circumstances, the *short-term* effect on potassium distribution is significant clinically. For example, when 5% dextrose is given i.v. in large volumes, the resulting elevation of insulin concentration can induce a rapid shift of potassium into the intracellular compartment, and consequently, a sharp fall in plasma potassium concentration. This effect has several potential clinical applications, and it must be considered when dextrose is given to patients who are already hypokalemic. In addition, i.v. potassium supplements given to raise plasma potassium levels should not be given in dextrose solution.

## Thyroxin

Thyroxin's presence is necessary in the embryonic chicken caprodeum for aldosterone to increase sodium transport (33). In toad bladder, it appears that thyroxin is primarily needed in the late (Na-independent) phase of sodium, potassium-ATPase activation (34). Amiloride-sensitive short-circuit current is also reduced in hypothyroidism (35). This may represent an interaction between aldosterone and thyroxin in cell signaling or transport.

## Acid –Base Disturbances

The distribution of potassium across cell membranes throughout the body is dependent on the electrochemical potential gradient for movement of potassium, the potassium conductance of the membrane, and the active transport of potassium by the sodium, potassium-ATPase. Changes in extracellular pH can affect these functions in several ways. When the concentration of hydrogen ion in the extracellular fluid increases, positively charged hydrogen ions enter the cell, and the electrochemical gradient favoring movement of potassium out of the cell is elevated. As a result, plasma potassium concentration increases to a variable degree with reductions in extracellular pH. The extent of the increase in potassium concentration associated with each 0.1-unit decrease in extracellular pH is usually, but not always, less than 0.2 to 0.4 mmol/L (36). In general, plasma potassium will increase to a greater extent when the reduction in pH is not accompanied by an accumulation of organic acids such as lactic acid and those associated with ketoacidosis. The explanation for this observation is not clear, however, it may be due to the ability of the organic anions to follow the hydrogen ions into the intracellular compartment, thereby preventing disturbance the electrochemical gradient governing potassium distribution.

Changes in plasma potassium concentration are less prominent in alkalosis than in acidosis, for unknown reasons.

## Exercise

During exercise skeletal muscle cells expend energy and deplete their stores of high energy phosphate compounds such as ATP. If the expenditure of

ATP is not greater than the rate at which the cell can replenish ATP by oxidative metabolism, the conditions that determine potassium distribution across the cell membrane may not be altered. But if the cell must perform anaerobic glycolysis to replenished ATP supplies, several membrane functions associated with potassium distribution will be affected. As ATP concentration at the cell membrane falls, its availability for the sodium, potassium-ATPase will be reduced and the rate of active transport of potassium into the cell will decline. In addition, ATP-sensitive potassium channels in the cell membrane will open in response to the reduced ATP concentration, permitting enhanced egress of potassium ions from the intracellular to the extracellular space. Consequently, when the muscle cells begin to shift to anaerobic metabolism, there is an increase in net flux of potassium into the extracellular fluid and into the venous blood draining the working muscle. Generally, arterial plasma potassium concentration increases minimally in exercise until the lactic acid concentration rises, signaling the onset of anaerobic metabolism in the working muscles (37). As exercise intensity increases, lactic acid concentration and potassium concentration will continue to rise, to as much as 2 mmol/L or more with exercise to exhaustion.

With cessation of exercise, cellular ATP concentration may rise very rapidly in recovering skeletal muscle cells, restoring the sodium, potassium-ATPase activity and the potassium conductance of the membrane to their original values. Potassium can be taken up at a high rate by skeletal muscle in first minutes of recovery. In this laboratory we analyzed the rate of change of potassium concentration in 13 subjects who ran on a treadmill to the point of exhaustion following a modified Bruce protocol (38). The changes in potassium concentration and epinephrine concentration are presented in Figure 2.4. Plasma potassium concentration rose during exercise from 3.98 to 5.09 mmol/L, and during recovery the concentration fell 0.54 mmol/L during the first minute, and 0.88 mmol/L during the first 2 minutes after treadmill exercise ended.

In one subject, potassium concentration fell from 5.26 to 4.33 mmol/L during the first minute, and further to 3.76 mmol/L during the second minute after exercise.

Epinephrine concentration increased during exercise from 63 to 497 pg/mL, and reached a maximum, 541 pg/mL, during the first minute of recovery when potassium concentration was falling rapidly. The combination of strongly elevated catecholamines and rapidly falling plasma potassium concentration may contribute to the vulnerability of the heart to serious arrhythmias in the first minutes immediately post-exercise.

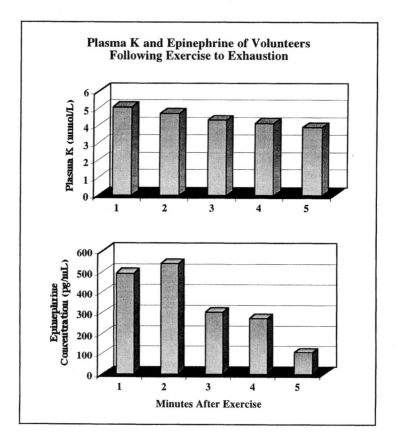

*Fig 2.4*

*Shown here are plasma K and epinephrine concentration data during the minutes following cessation of exhaustive treadmill exercise.  From reference 38.*

# LONG-TERM REGULATION OF POTASSIUM: IMPORTANCE OF ALDOSTERONE AND EXTRACELLULAR POTASSIUM CONCENTRATION

Aldosterone is actively and continuously involved in control of potassium balance and extracellular concentration, serving as a rapidly responsive effector in a negative feedback control system. As presented above, aldosterone stimulates secretion of potassium from the distal nephron, and alters the distribution of the ion across the cell membranes, shifting potassium into the cells from the extracellular fluid throughout the body. To integrate the findings from short-term *in vivo* and *in vitro* studies into an accurate understanding of how the potassium control system operates over long periods requires consideration of findings from experimental designs in which potassium regulation has been studied in intact animals over periods of several days or weeks. We conducted several series of such experiments in an effort to build an understanding of how the many possible components of the system function together over time.

## Regulation of Aldosterone Secretion by Extracellular Potassium Concentration.

Several factors are known to be capable of affecting aldosterone secretion from the zona glomerulosa of the adrenal cortex. Only two, however, respond to conditions associated with perturbations in potassium regulation: extracellular potassium concentration and the plasma concentration of angiotensin II. The individual stimulatory effects of each of these have been studied separately, and it is well accepted that they are prominent regulators of aldosterone secretion. However, the two stimuli vary simultaneously under most conditions associated with alterations in potassium balance. Therefore, we analyzed the interactions between them in stimulating aldosterone secretion (39). Angiotensin II and potassium were infused continuously so that three levels of angiotensin II and three levels of potassium administration were combined. The peptide infusion rates were 0, 5.0, and 10 ng/kg/min, and the potassium infusion rates were 0, 100, and

200 mmol/day. The plasma potassium and aldosterone concentrations were measured after 5 days and were plotted with plasma potassium concentration as the independent variable. The family of three curves, one for each level of angiotensin II infusion, is presented in Figure. 2.5, and normalized data from the same study are shown in three dimensions in Figure 2.6.

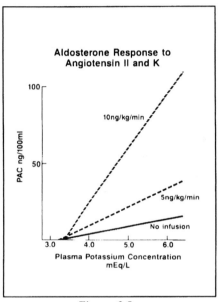

*Figure. 2.5*

*Interaction between angiotensin II and potassium in stimulating aldosterone secretion. Three rates of angiotensin II infusion, (0, 5, and 10 ng/kg/min) were combined with a range of potassium intakes for 5 day periods in groups of dogs. The two stimuli combine multiplicatively, with much greater stimulation by angiotensin II occurring at higher potassium concentrations than at lower levels of potassium. From reference 39.*

A striking multiplicative interaction between the two stimuli is apparent, the effect of higher angiotensin II levels rotating the relationship between potassium concentration and aldosterone levels upward and to the left around the same zero aldosterone point on the plasma potassium concentration axis (x-axis intercept). This type of interaction has several important physiological implications. For example, the sensitivity of aldosterone to a given change in concentration of one stimulus is a function of the concentration of the other; therefore, increasing angiotensin II concentration from normal to three times normal at a plasma potassium concentration of 4.5 mmol/L will result in a predicted increase in aldosterone from 1.2 to 3.7 times normal, whereas the same change in angiotensin II concentration at a plasma potassium concentration of 5.5 mmol/L will result in an increase from 2.2 to 6.7 times the normal aldosterone level.

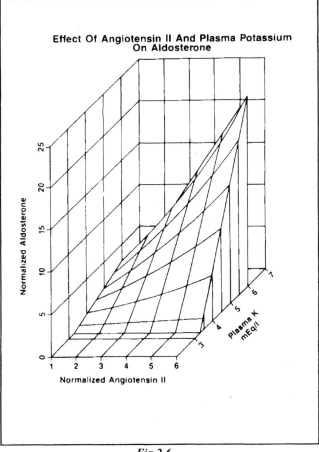

*Fig 2.6*

*Three dimensional representation of the interaction between angiotensin II and plasma potassium concentration in regulating plasma aldosterone concentration. Plasma angiotensin II and aldosterone concentrations are normalized, with 1.0 being the normal concentration.. From reference 39.*

The multiplicative interaction is of significant importance in understanding the regulation of aldosterone secretion under most normal physiological conditions as well as during experimental manipulations. We also analyzed the effect of time on the relationship between angiotensin II, potassium, and aldosterone secretion; measurements were recorded after 1, 2, and 5 days of combined angiotensin II and potassium intake levels. We found no change in the relationships over the 5-day period.

## Long-term Effects of Aldosterone on Potassium Excretion

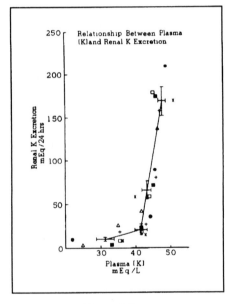

*Figure 2.7*

*Shown in the figure is the relationship between plasma potassium concentration and steady-state potassium excretion in adrenalectomized dogs maintained on a fixed, normal amount of aldosterone replacement. From reference 40.*

Changes in potassium concentration in the ECF can stimulate potassium secretion by the principal cells *in vitro*, and in short-term *in vivo* experiments. Over longer time courses, elevation of potassium concentration in the plasma and ECF also have been shown to be associated with increased rates of potassium excretion in rats and dogs. We observed that in adrenalectomized dogs given potassium intake ranging from 10 to 200 mmol/day while maintained on continuous replacement of a fixed, normal level of aldosterone, if the plasma potassium concentration were equal to or greater than the normal level, 4.2 mmol/L, each 0.1 mmol/L increase in plasma potassium concentration was associated with a 26 mmol/day increase in potassium excretion (40) (Figure 2.7); therefore, if plasma potassium concentration were initially 4.2 mmol/L and daily potassium excretion were 30 mmol/day, an increase in potassium concentration of 0.12 mmol/L would increase potassium excretion by 100%.

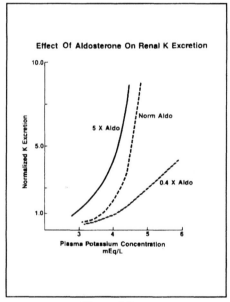

*Figure 2.8*

*Presented here are relationships between plasma potassium concentration and steady-state, normalized potassium excretion at three fixed levels of aldosterone, 0.4 normal, 1.0 normal, and 5 times normal. From reference 41.*

The magnitude of the slope of the relationship presented in Figure 2.7 suggests that the direct effect of ECF potassium concentration may be the most prominent controller of potassium excretion above the normal plasma concentration. However, below the normal intake level, the slope of the plasma potassium concentration -- urinary excretion relationship is much less impressive, 1.1 mmol/day per 0.1 mmol/L.

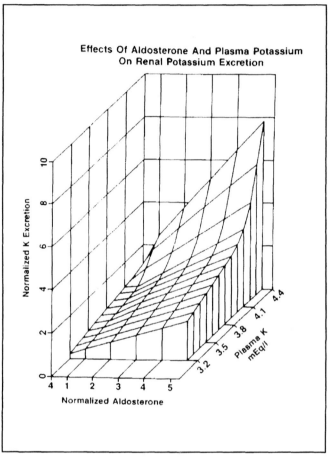

**Figure 2.9**

*Shown here is the three dimensional surface that describes the interaction between aldosterone (x axis) and plasma potassium concentration (z axis) in determining potassium excretion (y axis). Aldosterone and potassium excretion are normalized, with 1.0 being the normal value. From reference 41.*

We extended these studies to analyze the interaction of the kaliuretic effect of aldosterone with the powerful direct effect of ECF potassium concentration (41). Again, using adrenalectomized dogs that could be maintained on fixed levels of daily aldosterone replacement while potassium intake could be varied from 10 to 200 mmol/day, we analyzed the relationship between plasma potassium concentration and potassium excretion. The levels of aldosterone replacement used were from 40% to 500% of normal. The effect of aldosterone interacted multiplicatively with the direct effect of potassium concentration, shifting the relationship between plasma potassium concentration and potassium excretion upwards and to the left, as illustrated in Figure 2.8. The continuous interaction between aldosterone and potassium concentration is presented as a three dimensional surface in Figure 2.9, in which normalized aldosterone and plasma potassium concentration are plotted as the independent variables and normalized potassium excretion is shown as the dependent variable. Notice that the effect of aldosterone on excretion is greater as the concentration of plasma potassium increases to higher levels.

# SYSTEMS ANALYSES OF POTASSIUM REGULATION

The potassium control system has been studied in this laboratory using a nontraditional approach. Because the system is composed of several in-series and parallel interacting components, the operation of the system could not be analyzed by direct experimental techniques. Instead, a hypothesis concerning the structure and function of the control system was constructed and tested for validity. The hypothesis was put in the form of a mathematical model derived from a combination of new and existing concepts concerning operation of components of the potassium control system (42-44). In many cases, the equations related to the concepts were directly derived from the quantitative data obtained in experiments conducted in this laboratory. In others the equations were derived from information present in the literature.

The series of equations can be solved interatively using a digital computer in order to simulate the operation of the hypothetical control system in response to a variety of situations. By comparing the operation of the model system with experimental or clinical data, the validity of the hypothesis can be assessed. Such comparisons have been made, and to the present time the operation of the model has been in agreement with results of all of the numerous experimental manipulations with which it has been compared. Although agreement between model predictions and data does not represent an exclusive proof of the validity of the hypothesis, the consistent similarities between data and predictions in response to a wide range of challenges provide support for the hypotheses inherent in the model. With each subsequent case of agreement between simulations and experimental observation, the probability increases that the hypothetical control system closely corresponds to the long-term potassium control system. At this time no case of disagreement between simulations and experimental or clinical findings has been encountered.

## Model Predictions

The model together with the data describing the components of the system can be useful in understanding the relative magnitude of the importance of aldosterone and other components of the system in potassium regulation in a variety of conditions. Several will be discussed in the following paragraphs.

### Changes in Potassium Intake

When potassium intake increases, the system responds so that potassium excretion increases to match the level of intake within one to two days. With the initial increase in intake, the body retains potassium, since the rate of potassium excretion is below the rate of intake. As a result total body potassium and plasma potassium concentration begin to rise. This has the following two effects: stimulation of aldosterone secretion and a direct effect on the distal nephron to increase potassium excretion. The direct kaliuretic effects of the rising plasma potassium concentration along with the aldosterone effect elevate the rate of potassium excretion toward the rate of intake. However, a positive potassium balance will continue until the effects of plasma potassium concentration and aldosterone increase the potassium excretion rate to the intake rate. At the new balance point, plasma potassium concentration and aldosterone concentration will be elevated, and each will contribute to the increased rate of potassium excretion.

In an experiment conducted in this laboratory, potassium intake was increased in six normal dogs from 10 to 200 mmol/day. After 5 days, when the animals were again in a state of balance, plasma potassium concentration had risen from 4.29 ± 0.06 to 5.16 ± 0.12 mmol/L and aldosterone concentration rose from 4.4 ± 0.4 to 10.1 ± 2.1 ng/ml (39). The 20-fold increase in potassium excretion resulted primarily from the effects of these two factors. From the data presented in Figures 2.9, we can estimate that the 0.87 mmol/L increase in plasma potassium concentration, if acting alone, would increase steady-state potassium excretion to approximately 10.8 times above the initial level, whereas the 5.7 ng/ml or 2.3-fold increase in aldosterone concentration by itself would increase potassium excretion to approximately 3.5 times the initial level. Therefore, the plasma potassium concentration portion of the kaliuretic response to the 20-fold increase in potassium intake was the dominant factor, approximately three times as powerful as the aldosterone contribution. Although the aldosterone effect was of secondary importance, the two factors acting together in a multiplicative interaction were necessary to achieve the full 20-fold increase in excretion.

This example is typical of many experiments from this laboratory and others in which potassium intake has been altered while aldosterone and plasma potassium concentration have been measured carefully over periods of days. In the general case, in response to an increase in potassium intake, the rise in plasma potassium concentration is the dominant factor in increasing the rate of potassium excretion, the plasma concentration effect being approximately three times greater than the aldosterone effect. Under most physiological conditions involving changes in potassium intake, which lie well within the limits of the 20-fold change in potassium intake analyzed in the preceding example, the rise in potassium concentration is too small to stimulate large increases in aldosterone secretion, because the plasma potassium concentration increase is limited by the powerful kaliuretic effect of even small increases in the plasma concentration of potassium.

In experimental animals and in man, control of potassium concentration in the plasma is much more precise when potassium intake is raised above normal than it is when potassium intake falls below the normal level. In normal dogs consuming less than the normal level of intake, which is 30 mmol/day, even small decreases in intake are associated with relatively large decrements in plasma potassium concentration. Dogs can return to potassium balance on dietary intake of 10 mmol/day, or about one-third of the normal level of intake, although their level of plasma potassium may be reduced to approximately 3.2 to 3.4 mmol/L. Squires and Huth studied potassium conservation in normal male volunteers using three dietary levels of potassium intake: 25 to 27 mmol/day, 14 to 16 mmol/day, and 1 mmol/day (45). On the intake of 25 to 27 mmol/day (approximately one-third the normal level of intake) the subjects' urinary potassium excretion fell to the level of intake in four to seven days. On the intake of 14 to 16 mmol/day (1/5 to 1/4 normal) urinary excretion fell only to 19 to 27 mmol/day by the eighth day of the study. These subjects suffered a progressive potassium deficit that would have continued until their plasma potassium concentration fell to severely hypokalemic levels. Four subjects who received only one mmol/day of potassium sustained heavy losses of total body potassium. Three of these were able to decrease excretion to a level between 4 and 5 mmol/day. Cumulative loss reached 500 mmol in one patient after 21 days on one mmol/day intake. These studies demonstrate that potassium depletion can occur in normal subjects on daily rates of potassium intake of 25 to 27 mmol/day, and that potassium balance may possibly be achieved on a level of intake of 4 to 5 mmol/day, although not until a large potassium deficit and severe hypokalemia had been sustained.

**Change in Sodium Intake**

When sodium intake changes there is usually no change or only slight changes in potassium balance or in plasma potassium concentration, this in spite of the potentially powerful effect of sodium intake on potassium excretion described in Figure 2.2. When sodium intake increases, several components of the potassium control system interact to effectively regulate potassium balance. The increase in flow through the potassium-secreting portions of the nephron has a strong kaliuretic effect, and it has an effect on the renin release mechanism (46). Elevations in sodium intake are associated with reduced rates of renin release; the mechanism of the association is believed to be that an increase in flow or delivery of a component of the tubular fluid to the distal nephron results from the increase in sodium intake, and this change is sensed by the macula densa. The macula densa in turn provides an inhibitory signal to the renin-release mechanism in the juxtaglomerular cells of the afferent arteriole. At the time that a kaliuretic increase in flow through the potassium secreting portions of the nephron begins, renin release also begins to fall. As renin release and angiotensin II concentration fall, so does the rate of aldosterone secretion. Therefore, the same factor that has the kaliuretic potential, the increase in distal flow rate, also imparts an indirect but simultaneous signal to the zona glomerulosa to reduce aldosterone secretion, thereby providing an antikaliuretic influence on the distal nephron, and counterbalancing the effect of the increase in flow rate.

In a study of potassium regulation during changes in sodium intake conducted here, sodium intake was increased from 10 to 200 mmol/day in a group of 12 dogs (47). There were no measurable changes in either plasma potassium concentration, which remained approximately 4.0 mmol/L, or in daily potassium excretion rate (approximately 25 mmol/day) in response to the 20-fold increase in sodium intake. However, plasma renin activity fell from $1.1 \pm 0.2$ to $0.4 \pm 0.1$ ng/ml/hr, and plasma aldosterone concentration fell from $12.9 \pm 1.5$ to $8.0 \pm 1.3$ ng/100 ml (normal value for that assay was 10.6 ng/100 ml). In response to the increase in sodium intake and flow/delivery to the macula densa, renin release fell, resulting in a 67% fall in plasma renin activity and a 40% fall in aldosterone concentration. The predicted effect of such a fall in aldosterone acting alone on potassium excretion at a plasma potassium concentration of 4.0 mmol/L would be a 50% decrease (Figure 2.9), while the estimated effect of the increase in sodium intake from 10 to 200 mmol/day acting alone at a plasma concentration of 4.0 mmol/L would be an increase in potassium excretion of 176% (Figure 2.2). Apparently the multiplicative interaction between the two effects acting in opposition resulted in no change in potassium excretion in response to the 20-fold increase in sodium intake.

The importance of the fall in aldosterone concentration in potassium regulation during increases in sodium intake was vividly apparent in a companion study carried out with the one described above (47). Again, sodium intake was raised from 10 to 200 mmol/day in a group of dogs, but in this case they were adrenalectomized and received a continuous infusion of aldosterone at a constant rate (100 micrograms/day) throughout the study; therefore, aldosterone concentration could not be adjusted in response to the increase in sodium intake.

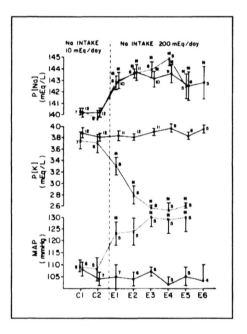

**Figure 2.10**

*Shown in the figure are plasma sodium and potassium concentrations, and mean arterial pressure data from an intact group of dogs (solid lines) and an adrenalectomized group that received fixed aldosterone replacement. After two days of control measurements (C1 and C2) sodium intake was increased from 10 to 200 mEq/day while data were collected for an additional six days (E1 through E6). The elevation of sodium intake resulted in a dramatic fall in plasma potassium concentration in the animals with fixed aldosterone concentration. From reference 47.*

In this condition the same 20-fold increase in sodium intake resulted in a 31% fall in plasma potassium concentration from $3.71 \pm 0.15$ to $2.51 \pm 0.04$ mmol/L and a kaliuresis that lasted until it was checked by the profound hypokalemia, as shown in Figure 2.10. In the absence of feedback control of aldosterone, potassium regulation was ineffective during the change in sodium intake. When the system is intact, the renin release mechanism responds rapidly to the change in flow into the distal nephron and signals a decrease in aldosterone secretion apparently before a significant increase in potassium excretion can occur. The highly effective manner in which potassium control is maintained during large changes in sodium intake that have the potential to severely alter potassium excretion demonstrates that the components of the system respond rapidly, and that the responses of the different components of the system are very well matched. For the system to work as well as it does, a given increase in flow into the distal nephron must result in a decrease in aldosterone concentration that will exactly offset the kaliuretic effect of the increase in flow. However, between the increase in flow and the change in aldosterone concentration are two functions; one relating flow past the macula densa to renin release, and the other relating angiotensin II concentration and aldosterone secretion. The functions describing the control of the secretion of these factors are nonlinear, and the functions describing the effects of sodium intake and aldosterone on potassium excretion are complex and interactive with related variables. The interrelationships among the components are such that when the system is intact, it is remarkably effective in controlling potassium excretion and plasma potassium concentration (43).

**Potassium Regulation Over Ranges of Sodium and Potassium Intake**

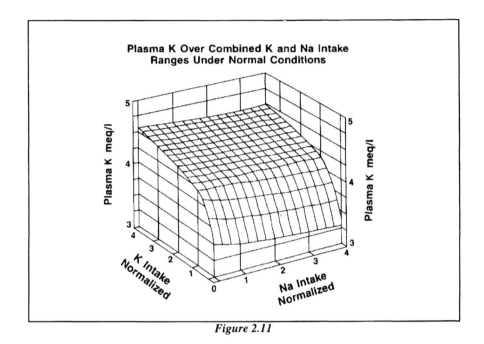

*Figure 2.11*

*Presented in the figure is the three dimensional surface representing regulation of plasma potassium concentration during combined sodium and potassium intakes ranging from 0.25 to 4.0 normal rates. From reference 43.*

In previous portions of this section, analyses were presented concerning responses of the system that regulates potassium to changes in either sodium intake, potassium intake, or aldosterone levels. Under many physiological conditions two or three of these variables change simultaneously. A graphical analysis of simulated potassium regulation in response to a range of combined changes in sodium and potassium intake is presented in Figure 2.11. Normalized sodium and potassium intakes are both plotted as independent variables along the bases of the figure and plasma potassium concentration is presented in the vertical direction. The intake scales are normalized, 1.0 being the normal rate of intake, or 100% of normal. The range of intakes analyzed extends from 0.25 to 4.0 normal with values presented in increments of 0.25 normalized units. In essence, the surface represents the control of plasma potassium concentration in response to a range of simulated combined sodium and potassium intakes.

Several features of the surface are noteworthy. First, the surface is nearly flat above the normal level of potassium intake (1.0 on the potassium intake axis), which indicates that regulation of plasma potassium concentration is excellent above the normal level of potassium intake. Going from the point of normal rates of potassium and sodium intake (1.0 on both the potassium and sodium intake axes) to the point of 4.0 normal potassium intake and 1.0 normal sodium intake results in a change in plasma potassium concentration from 4.20 to 4.60 mmol/L (a 10% increase in concentration over a 400% increase in intake). The increase in potassium excretion that returned the system to a point of balance at the higher level of potassium intake resulted from: 1) the direct effect of the rise in plasma potassium concentration on renal potassium excretion, and 2) from the kaliuretic effect of a predicted increase in aldosterone levels from 1.00 to 1.34 normal, stimulated by the hyperkalemia. Moving along the sodium intake axis from the point of normal sodium and potassium intake to the point of normal potassium intake and 4.0 normal sodium intake results in a decrease in plasma potassium concentration from 4.20 to 4.09 mmol/L due to the change in plasma potassium and the predicted reduction in aldosterone to 0.67 of normal. Control below the normal level of potassium intake is less precise than control in response to excess potassium intake. Again, starting from the point of normal sodium and potassium intakes and moving along the potassium intake axis to the point of 0.25 potassium intake and normal sodium intake results in a fall in plasma potassium concentration from 4.20 to 3.45 mmol/L (an 18% decrease in response to a 4-fold decrease in potassium intake), in spite of a predicted fall in aldosterone to 0.57 of normal. This impaired control effectiveness results mainly from the decrease in sensitivity of the renal response to changes in plasma potassium concentration below 4.20 mmol/L (Figure 2.7). However, as long as plasma potassium concentration is above this level, as it is over most of the surface when potassium intake is normal or above normal, plasma potassium regulation is excellent in response to a wide range of combined sodium and potassium intakes.

Aldosterone's precise role in potassium regulation can be visually assessed by comparing the surface describing simulated potassium control by the normal system shown in Figure 2.11 with the surface describing simulated potassium control with feedback control of aldosterone secretion blocked, which is shown in Figure 2.12.

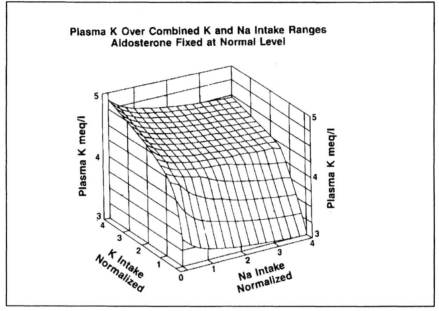

*Figure 2.12*

*Presented in the figure is the three dimensional surface representing regulation of plasma potassium concentration during combined sodium and potassium intakes ranging from 0.25 to 4.0 normal rates, but with simulated aldosterone concentration held constant at the level observed with normal combined sodium and potassium intakes. From reference 43*

The simulations used to generate the surfaces were identical except that in this case the aldosterone level was held constant at the normal level, 1.0; consequently, in response to the simulated changes in electrolyte intake, the system could not alter the aldosterone level. Therefore, the difference between the two surfaces is due to the effects of aldosterone on potassium regulation.

There are both important differences as well as similarities between the surfaces. The differences can be seen in regions in which the Na-to-K intake ratio is greatly different from 1.0. For example, when sodium intake is below normal and potassium intake is greater than normal, the surface in Figure 2.12 slopes upward, whereas in Figure 2.11, which describes the behavior of the intact system, the same region of the surface remains flat. At the extreme point at which sodium intake is 0.25 and potassium intake is 4.0 (Na:K = 1/16) plasma potassium concentration on the intact surface is 4.64 mmol/L, while on the surface in which aldosterone levels are fixed the plasma potassium concentration value is 4.95 mmol/L. However, there are large regions of the two surfaces that are nearly identical. In general, this area covers the region in which the Na:K intake ratio is between approximately 0.3 and 3.0. On the normal surface at the point at which sodium intake is 1.5 normal and potassium intake is 4.0 normal, the value for plasma potassium concentration is 4.51 mmol/L, and on the surface without feedback control of aldosterone, the plasma potassium concentration value at the same point is 4.56 mmol/L. At the point where sodium intake is 4.0 and potassium intake is 1.5 normal the plasma potassium concentration for the intact and constant aldosterone surfaces again are similar, 4.28 and 4.22 mmol/L, respectively. Therefore, over the range of intake combinations normally encountered, feedback control of aldosterone is of minor importance for precise control of plasma potassium concentration. Other mechanisms, especially the direct effects of changes in plasma potassium concentration on potassium excretion, respond to changes in intake combinations in a manner that provides adequate regulation of potassium excretion in the absence of changes in aldosterone levels. Only when the intake combinations are extreme does active participation of the aldosterone feedback mechanism significantly improve the precision of potassium regulation.

## SUMMARY

On the basis of the present analysis, one may concluded that aldosterone is a major component of the system that regulates potassium over long time periods. The hormone's participation in the control system is regulated by the multiplicative interaction of the two stimuli of aldosterone secretion, angiotensin II and plasma potassium concentration. The most prominent regulator of potassium excretion is the direct effect of changes in extracellular potassium concentration on secretion of the ion into the distal nephron. This mechanism is approximately three times as powerful as the aldosterone effect in increasing potassium excretion in response to increases in the rate of potassium intake. Aldosterone participates in control of the distribution of potassium between the intra- and extracellular spaces, a greater proportion of total body potassium being within the cells at higher levels of aldosterone. The shift in distribution can be large so that plasma potassium concentration may fall by 1.0 mmol/L or more with only small change in potassium excretion in response to a several fold increase in aldosterone concentration.

Aldosterone's most prominent function in potassium regulation is in preventing changes in potassium excretion during changes in sodium excretion. Increases in flow through the potassium-secreting portion of the distal nephron strongly augment potassium secretion. However, as distal flow increases, for example following an increase in sodium intake, aldosterone secretion decreases as a result of a reduction in renin release and angiotensin II concentration; the reduced aldosterone concentration offsets the kaliuretic influence of the increase in flow rate, so that in general, no change in potassium balance occurs. Aldosterone is not the most powerful component of the systems regulating potassium and excretion, but the aldosterone component is the only mechanism that enables the system to simultaneously maintain balance of both potassium and sodium over wide combined ranges of intakes of the two ions.

# Chapter 3

# INTERACTIONS BETWEEN CARDIOVASCULAR PHARMACOTHERAPEUTICS AND POTASSIUM REGULATION

## DIURETICS

## ANGIOTENSIN CONVERTING ENZYME INHIBITORS AND ANGIOTENSIN II RECEPTOR ANTAGONISTS

## MINERALOCORTICOID ANTAGONISTS

## BETA ADRENERGIC RECEPTOR ANTAGONISTS

## SUMMARY

Control of potassium is accomplished by regulating the rate of secretion of potassium from the principal cells located in the distal nephron and collecting tubules. Several of the most commonly used medications for hypertension and heart failure affect either glomerular filtration rate or sodium reabsorption in portions of the tubules proximal to the potassium secreting regions, thereby affecting conditions that determine potassium flux from the principal cells to the tubular lumen. Consequently, medications whose primary functions are to reduce extracellular fluid volume or reduce vascular resistance, have significant impacts on potassium excretion and long-term control of potassium. Diuretics, mineralocorticoid antagonists, angiotensin converting enzyme inhibitors and angiotensin II receptor antagonists, and beta blockers -- some of the most commonly used medications in cardiovascular medicine -- all interact with the system that regulates potassium excretion. Table 3.1 lists commonly prescribed medications that can in some cases affect potassium regulation.

*Table 3.1*
*Medications That Affect Potassium Regulation*

| REDUCE PLASMA K | INCREASE PLASMA K |
| --- | --- |
| loop diuretics | mineralocorticoid antagonists |
| thiazide diuretics | ang II receptor antagonists |
| penicillin derivatives | ACE inhibitors |
| amphotericin B | Beta adrenergic antagonists |
| mineralocorticoid agonists | digitalis |
| insulin | |
| beta adrenergic agonists | |
| mannitol | |

# DIURETICS

All diuretics affect potassium excretion. Those that act in the proximal tubule, the ascending limb of the loop of Henle and in the early portions of the distal nephron inhibit absorption of sodium from the tubular fluid, and lead indirectly to elevation of potassium excretion from more distal portions of the tubule. Potassium-sparing diuretics inhibit potassium secretion from the principal cells of the distal nephron by opposing the actions of aldosterone or by blocking sodium exchange across the luminal membrane of the principal cells.

Loop diuretics -- furosemide, bumetanide and ethycrinic acid -- strongly inhibit sodium reabsorption in the ascending limb of the loop of Henle. They act by competing for the chloride site on the sodium - potassium - 2 chloride cotransport mechanism in the luminal membrane of the cells of the ascending limb. Thiazide compounds appear to inhibit sodium-chloride cotransport in the apical membrane of cells of the early portions of the distal nephron. Carbonic anhydrase inhibitors block sodium reabsorption associated with bicarbonate absorption in the proximal tubule. The actions of these three types of diuretics inhibit sodium reabsorption, increasing the sodium concentration and the rate of flow in the potassium secreting portions of the late distal, connecting, and initial collecting tubules. Increase in sodium concentration in the tubular fluid can stimulate potassium diffusion from the principal cells into the lumen by two mechanisms (48,49): first, the sodium gradient from lumen to cell favors entry of sodium ions, thereby creating a diffusion potential that can offset the potassium diffusion potential created as potassium ions move from cell to lumen; second, entry of sodium ions into the principal cell raises intracellular sodium concentration, stimulating the sodium, potassium-ATPase in the basolateral membrane, which elevates the rate of potassium uptake from the extracellular fluid. The increased rate of flow associated with loop and thiazide diuretics elevates potassium excretion by attenuating a rise in potassium concentration in the tubular fluid as potassium ions diffuse from the principal cells into the lumen; consequently, the concentration gradient favoring diffusion of potassium from cell to lumen is not limited by accumulation of potassium ions in the tubular fluid.

In addition to their tubular effect on potassium excretion, loop diuretics and thiazides also indirectly stimulate secretion of aldosterone. Reduction in extracellular fluid volume resulting from diuretic administration will tend to increase the activity of the renin-angiotensin-aldosterone system. Elevated aldosterone levels stimulate potassium secretion by the principal cells, interacting multiplicatively with the kaliuretic actions elicited by the diuretics at the tubular level.

Use of thiazide and loop diuretics will tend to induce a mild alkalosis that can exacerbate hypokalemia. The diuretics promote an equimolar loss of sodium and chloride along with water, leaving behind in the contracted extracellular fluid volume an unchanged quantity of bicarbonate ions. The alkalosis is characterized by an elevated bicarbonate ion concentration along with less than normal chloride concentration. Additional loss of hydrogen ions from the extracellular fluid may result from stimulation of hydrogen ion secretion by the distal nephron by elevated aldosterone concentration associated with the secondary effects of the diuretics. An intracellular shift of potassium ions associate with the alkalosis may contribute as much as 0.4 mmol/L decrease in extracellular potassium concentration per 0.1 unit increase in extracellular pH to the hypokalemia induced by the diuretics (36,50).

While thiazides and loop diuretics promote a significant increase in potassium excretion, the degree and hypokalemia and potassium depletion resulting from their use varies from patient to patient. The lower the initial plasma potassium concentration and the initial level of potassium intake, the greater the risk that the patient will become significantly hypokalemic. The level of sodium intake can affect the kaliuretic response to diuretics, with greater potassium loss being associated with higher levels of sodium intake. Similarly, the diuretic response affects the magnitude of potassium loss; for example, patients who have a large quantity of edema fluid that can be mobilized by the diuretic will tend to have a greater potassium loss along with their greater fluid volume loss than non-edematous patients with hypertension, who respond with only a modest diuresis. The initial level of activity of the renin-angiotensin-aldosterone system also is important in determining the potassium loss associated with diuretics. Patients with high initial levels of activity will respond to diuretic-induced volume depletion with even higher rates of renin release, aldosterone secretion and potassium loss. The duration of treatment and especially the dosage of diuretic are important factors that affect development of a state of potassium depletion. If hydrochlorothiazide is used to treat essential hypertension, the incidence of hypokalemia is dose related, increasing from 25% with 50 mg per day to 40 to 50% with 100 mg per day (51-53). Chlorthalidone, which is longer acting, is even more likely to produce hypokalemia.

Potassium-sparing diuretics act on the segments of the distal tubule and collecting duct that secrete potassium. Amiloride and triamterene both interfere with the sodium conductive pathway in the apical membrane of the principal cells (54). The net effects of these drugs on the pattern of renal electrolyte excretion are similar: reduced sodium reabsorption and decreased potassium and hydrogen ion secretion. Combining these agents with diuretics that act more proximally can be effective in attenuating potassium loss and development of alkalosis. Using potassium sparing diuretics or spironolactone without concomitant thiazide or loop diuretics will result in potassium retention and elevation of plasma potassium concentration that may be significant if the patient has a high level of potassium intake, is taking potassium supplements, or has compromised renal function.

# ANGIOTENSIN CONVERTING ENZYME INHIBITORS AND ANGIOTENSIN II RECEPTOR ANTAGONISTS

Interruption of the function of the renin-angiotensin system by converting enzyme inhibitors or angiotensin II receptor blocking agents can alter the functions of several elements in the potassium control system (55). Reducing angiotensin II concentration or effect inhibits reabsorption of sodium in the proximal tubule resulting in an initial increase in delivery of sodium and tubular fluid to the distal nephron. This early effect results in a kaliuresis that can only be seen within the first few hours following intravenous administration of converting enzyme inhibitors. Over longer periods of time, reduction in angiotensin II concentration results in reduced rate of secretion of aldosterone from the zona glomerulosa of the adrenal gland. As plasma aldosterone concentration falls, the aldosterone-induced functions of the principal cells become less active, and the rate of potassium secretion declines. Over a period of days, potassium retention will lead to elevation of plasma potassium concentration, which will have a stimulatory effect on aldosterone secretion. In time, a new state of balance will be achieved, characterized by plasma potassium concentration being somewhat higher than the initial level, and plasma aldosterone concentration being lower than the initial value. The magnitude of the increase in potassium concentration will depend on several factors, including initial concentration of potassium, the initial level of activity of the renin-angiotensin-aldosterone system, the level of daily sodium and potassium intake, and renal function.

For the vast majority of patients with normal renal function, hyperkalemia is not a significant problem associated with use of converting enzyme inhibitors or angiotensin II receptor blocking agents, unless the patients are taking potassium supplements or potassium-sparing diuretics (56,57).

Generally, the degree of increase in plasma potassium concentration associated with converting enzyme inhibition and angiotensin II receptor antagonists will be inversely related to the glomerular filtration rate. However, renal function and glomerular filtration rate frequently improve with converting enzyme inhibitors, especially when the reduced state of renal function is secondary to inadequate cardiac output. Interestingly, Dzau et al. reported that treatment of patients with severe congestive heart failure (NYHA Class IV) with converting enzyme inhibitors for six weeks reduced plasma potassium concentration from borderline hyperkalemic levels ($4.8 \pm 0.2$ mmol/L) to normal ($4.3 \pm 0.2$), in association with marked increases in cardiac and renal function (creatinine clearance increased from $19.7 \pm 3.0$ to $33.3 \pm 6.3$ mL/min) (58). The fall in potassium concentration occurred in spite of a reduction in plasma aldosterone concentration from $65 \pm 14$ to $16 \pm 4$ ng/dL. This example illustrates the significance of the interplay between tubular flow rate, which can be strongly influenced by changes in renal hemodynamics, and the effect of aldosterone on the principal cells. In this case, the improvement of GFR and the attending kaliuretic effect of elevated rate of distal delivery of tubular fluid more than off-set the antikaliuretic effect of the reduction in aldosterone concentration.

## MINERALOCORTICOID ANTAGONISTS

Spironolactone is an aldosterone antagonist that blocks the effects of the hormone on the principal cells of the tubule. As a result, the sodium conductance in the apical membrane is reduced, and the activity and number of sodium, potassium-ATPase in the basolateral membrane is reduced. Therefore, spironolactone provides the clinically attractive combination of natriuresis and diuresis without kaliuresis. The magnitude of the natriuresis and diuresis is modest compared to that of loop diuretics, because the amount of sodium remaining in the tubule at the end of the distal nephron is only about 2% of the filtered amount, versus 15 to 20% in the ascending limb of the loop of Henle where the loop diuretics act. However, the natriuresis and diuresis persist over a much longer period than those of the thiazides and loop diuretics. Spironolactone was first introduced in 1972, and in trials its efficacy was found to be comparable to the that of thiazides for treatment of hypertension and congestive heart failure (59). Acceptance of spironolactone was limited by several factors. First, it was more expensive than thiazide diuretics. Second, its onset of action was slow compared to that of loop diuretics or thiazides. When first administered, little effect or clinical improvement is observed. However, over a period of weeks as the natriuresis continues, the impact on the fluid volume and cardiovascular status of the patient becomes more and more significant. This is in contrast to the rapid onset of action of diuretics that act in more proximal portions of the tubule, although loop and thiazide diuretics do not produce additional sodium loss after the first week of administration. Third, spironolactone was associated with dose-dependent antiandrogenic side effects, especially in the 50 to 100 mg daily dose employed when the compound was first introduced. The gynecomastia in men and menstrual disturbances in women proved to be intolerable for many patients. More recently, smaller doses, 12.5 to 25 mg/day, have been found to be efficacious and produce a lower incidence of side effects.

When given alone, spironolactone can cause a sufficient quantity of potassium retention to lead to hyperkalemia. The risk of hyperkalemia is inversely related to the dose, and directly related to the level of potassium intake. Currently, however, spironolactone is usually given in combination with a loop or thiazide diuretic in a dosage adjusted to offset the kaliuresis associated with the increased rate of flow to the distal portion of the nephron.

Recently, spironolactone has attracted intense attention following the outcome of the RALES trial, in which addition of 25 mg per day of spironolactone to standard therapy for severe congestive heart failure significantly increased cardiac function and survival (60). In nearly all patients spironolactone was combined with a converting enzyme inhibitor and a loop diuretic. In this group, whose initial plasma creatinine concentration was less than 2.5 mg/dL, the investigators reported that plasma potassium concentration increased by 0.3 mmol/L, and severe hyperkalemia was reported in only 2% of the treated subjects.

## BETA ADRENERGIC RECEPTOR ANTAGONISTS

Epinephrine is associated with beta-2 receptor mediated potassium uptake by skeletal muscle that appears to protect against exercised induced hyperkalemia (23,37). During conditions of the emotional stress not associated with exercise, such as an intense emotional arousal, pain, trauma, or myocardial infarction, activation of the sympathetic nervous system can result in transfer of potassium from the extracellular fluid into the cells of the muscles in sufficient quantity to reduce transiently potassium concentration by 1.0 mmol/L or more. If beta adrenergic antagonists are used chronically for treatment of hypertension or other cardiovascular diseases, these effects to transiently alter potassium distribution will be attenuated. However, the beta adrenergic antagonists have little impact on long-term potassium regulation, and consequently, their clinical application is rarely associated with significant hyperkalemia.

## SUMMARY

Commonly used medications for hypertension and heart failure affect either glomerular filtration rate or sodium reabsorption in portions of the tubules proximal to the potassium secreting regions, thereby affecting conditions that determine potassium flux from the principal cells to the tubular lumen. As a result, potassium depletion and hypokalemia are common complications associated with treatment of these diseases.

# Chapter 4

# POTASSIUM DEPLETION AND HYPOKALEMIA

### SYMPTOMS

### ETIOLOGY

### DIAGNOSIS

### TREATMENT

### SUMMARY

Potassium depletion and hypokalemia are defined clinically as reduction in total body potassium of approximately 8%, and reduction in plasma potassium concentration from the normal value of 4.2 to 3.5 mmol/L. Below these levels, symptoms may begin to occur that are directly attributable to the change in potassium status. The potassium content of the human body is approximately 50 mmol/kg, with skeletal and cardiac muscle having 70 to 75 mmol/kg, and adipose cells having very little potassium. Under steady state conditions, plasma concentration usually varies directly with total body potassium, with approximately a 10% change in total potassium being associated 1.0 mmol/L change in plasma concentration (18). However, as noted previously, changes in plasma potassium concentration may result from transfer of potassium into or out of the cellular compartment. Hypokalemia that persists for periods of days is most often associated with depletion of total potassium content, due either to inadequate intake or excessive loss of potassium from the G.I. tract, the skin, or from the kidneys.


# SYMPTOMS

A significant percentage of the population of industrialized cultures consumes diets low in potassium content throughout their lives. Most subjects who are taking in 25 to 60 mmol/day will have plasma concentrations between 3.5 to 4.2 mmol/L, will excrete 20 to 55 mmol/day, and will have no acute symptoms of potassium depletion, unless they are challenged by a circumstance that increases their rate of potassium loss or reduces their level of intake (for review see reference 61). Patients with plasma levels between 2.5 and 3.0 mmol/L may have symptoms related specifically to their hypokalemia and potassium depletion. In these, most often potassium deficiency is severe and is associated with voluminous diarrhea, ingestion of two different classes of diuretics, treatment for diabetic ketoacidosis, malnutrition resulting from eating disorders or alcoholism, strenuous physical work in hot environments with high rates of sweating, or the potassium deficiency may result from renal tubular acidosis. Symptoms are initially vague and may be described as lack of vigor, weakness, fatigue-associated restlessness, muscular discomfort, and occasionally, exercise-induced muscle cramps. Severe potassium deficiency occurring rapidly may result in severe weakness or frank paralysis. In spite of the muscular weakness, deep tendon reflexes are retained. Severe muscle pain, tenderness, and weakness suggest development of rhabdomyolysis. Symptoms will be inversely proportional to the level of potassium concentration, and will occur at higher levels of potassium in the presence of hypernatremia. Rapidly developing potassium depletion will elicit symptoms at higher levels of plasma concentration than in patients in whom hypokalemia develops over periods of months. Rhabdomyolosis due to potassium depletion may occur in healthy persons who have become gradually potassium depleted due to heat stress, and then undertake exhaustive physical exercise.

Muscle weakness and paralysis induced by hypokalemia usually do not occur above plasma concentrations of 2.5 mmol/L. While an acute reduction in extracellular potassium concentration would be expected to hyperpolarize the cell membrane potential, long-term hypokalemia is associated with depolarization of the membrane potential of skeletal muscle cells from the usual resting level of -86 mV to -50 to -55 mV. Presumably, this depolarization is related to an increase in sodium conductance and/or a decrease in potassium conductance. If the membrane potential rises above the threshold level of about -65 mV, the muscle cells become refractory and an action potential cannot be generated. This is the case in severe, prolonged potassium depletion when the resting potential of skeletal muscle approaches or exceeds the threshold potential. Initially, muscle weakness may be noted, which may progress to paralysis. Typically, the muscles of the lower extremities are affected first, particularly the quadriceps. In severe cases the muscles of the trunk and upper extremities become impaired, and eventually respiration become affected. Death may ensue from respiratory failure. Involvement of smooth muscle in the gastrointestinal tract can produce symptoms of abdominal distention, anorexia, vomiting, constipation, and paralytic ilieus (62).

Rhabdomyolysis, muscle cramps, tenderness, and atrophy may be seen in patients with severe potassium depletion. These effects may be due to inhibition of enzymes associated with cellular metabolism by potassium depletion, or the cellular effects may be secondary to relative ischemia associated with impaired blood flow regulation to the muscle during exercise (63-65).

As deficiency becomes severe, creatine kinase (CK) activity in serum may become detectable. Frank rhabdomyolysis will result in marked elevation of CK; in addition, serum aldolase activity, serum glutamic oxaloactetic transaminase (SGOT), and lactic dehydrogenase all may be elevated (66).

Several aspects of renal function are altered by potassium depletion that is the consequence of inadequate intake or extrarenal loss of potassium (for review see reference 67). The inability to form a concentrated urine develops gradually as plasma potassium approaches 3.0 mmol/L, and is due to reduced responsiveness of the collecting tubule epithelium to vasopressin. However, because maximal urine concentration remains above 300 mosm/kg during potassium depletion, the degree of polyuria is typically mild compared to that of central diabetes insipidus.

Ammonia production by the renal tubular cells is increased in hypokalemia due to intracellular acidosis that accompanies a shift of potassium ions out of the cells and entry of hydrogen ions in exchange. Consequently, ammonium and hydrogen ion excretion in the urine are elevated in potassium depletion. The intracellular acidosis and elevated hydrogen ion concentration in the tubular fluid also promote bicarbonate reabsorption that may contribute to metabolic alkalosis.

Tubular absorption of sodium during potassium depletion appears to be stimulated. Potassium depleted patients have a relative inability to excrete a sodium load, which can lead to sodium retention and edema in patients consuming a high sodium, low potassium intake.

Ability to conserve potassium persists in potassium depletion resulting from extrarenal causes; patients with potassium depletion associated with inadequate intake or excessive G.I. tract losses will have potassium excretion of 25 mmol/day or less.

Hyperglycemia associated with Type II diabetes mellitus may be exacerbated by thiazide diuretic induced hypokalemia. The effect may be due to both an inhibition of insulin secretion and a reduction in insulin sensitivity (68). It has been reported that both are improved in thiazide treated type II diabetics by correction of potassium depletion (68).

The cardiac symptoms associated with potassium depletion will be presented separately in a later chapter.

# ETIOLOGY OF POTASSIUM DEPLETION AND HYPOKALEMIA

*Table 3.1*
*Causes of hypokalemia*

| |
|---|
| Inadequate intake |
| Excessive renal loss |
|       Mineralocorticoid excess |
|            Primary hyperaldosteronism |
|            Cushing's syndrome |
|            Congenital adrenal hyperplasia |
|            Hyperreninism |
|            Bartter's syndrome |
|            Exogenous mineralocorticoids |
|       Excessive flow to the distal nephron |
|            Diuretics |
|            High sodium intake |
|       Nonreabsorbable anions in the distal tubular fluid |
|            Metabolic Acidosis |
|            Type I and II renal tubular acidosis |
|            Diabetic ketoacidosis |
|            Penicillin derivatives |
| Gastrointestinal loss |
| Loss in Sweat |

Hypokalemia is defined as plasma potassium concentration less than 3.5 mmol/L. Under normal, steady-state conditions, plasma potassium concentration varies directly with total body potassium content, and for potassium in the plasma to fall from the normal level, 4.2 mmol/L, to hypokalemic levels requires a reduction in total body potassium content of about 7 to 8% from the normal content of 3500 mmol in a 70 kg man (18). Hypokalemia and potassium depletion are not uncommon, especially in subgroups that are at high risk for development of cardiovascular disease. Long-term depletion can result from either inadequate intake or excessive loss of potassium from the G.I. tract, the skin through sweat, or from the kidneys. Transiently, hypokalemia can follow from a shift from the extracellular compartment into the cells. The causes of hypokalemia and potassium depletion are outlined in Table 3.1.

## Inadequate Intake

The average dietary potassium content of inhabitants of Western cultures is approximately 60 to 80 mmol/day (4). Recall from Chapter 2 that plasma potassium concentration is well regulated in response to increases in potassium intake above the normal level; however, if intake is reduced below normal, plasma potassium concentration will fall before potassium excretion decreases to the level of intake. Furthermore, if a greater than normal level of sodium intake is combined with sub-normal potassium intake, the fall in potassium concentration will be exacerbated (Figure 2.2 and 2.3).

The kidney's ability to conserve potassium is not as effective as its ability to limit sodium excretion. The minimum daily rate of potassium excretion is approximately 5 to 10 mmol/day, but this level of excretion is not reached for more than several weeks of exposure to a nearly potassium-free diet, after severe potassium depletion and hypokalemia have developed. When potassium intake initially falls, renal excretion of potassium continues at the initial rate until the functions of several elements of the control system respond to the lower level of intake. As the rate of excretion exceeds the rate of intake, a negative potassium balance begins to accumulate, and in a short time plasma potassium concentration will begin to fall. From the decline in concentration of potassium in the plasma will follow a reduction in aldosterone secretion, and as a consequence, potassium secretory functions of the principal cells of the distal nephron and collecting duct will decline. In addition, the reduction in extracellular potassium concentration will affect directly potassium secretion from the principal cells by decreasing the rate of activity of the sodium, potassium-ATPase in the basolateral membrane of the cells. In time, these responses to the reduced rate of intake will lower the rate of potassium excretion to the new rate of intake. However, the compensatory responses all are triggered by negative potassium balance and reductions in plasma potassium concentration. Therefore, balance on a reduced rate of potassium intake will not occur without some degree of potassium depletion and reduction in plasma concentration. And, the greater the reduction in intake, the greater will be the reduction in total body potassium and plasma level before balance is restored.

The level of sodium intake has an significant effect on the response to potassium restriction. With high levels of sodium intake, the rate of flow through the potassium-secreting portions of the nephron is elevated, which is kaliuretic. Therefore, with higher rates of sodium intake, more intense compensatory measures must be achieved in order to regain potassium balance following a reduction in intake, more intense measures that must be elicited by greater degrees of potassium depletion and reduction in plasma concentration. In the southeastern portion of the United States the African-American population consumes a diet containing on the average 20 to 40 mmol/day of potassium together with very high levels of sodium intake (3,5). This habitual combination of low potassium with high sodium places a large portion of the group at risk of living in a state of moderate potassium depletion. And it is this group that has a high relative risk of all major cardiovascular diseases, including hypertension, coronary artery disease, stroke, cardiac hypertrophy, and congestive heart failure.

## Excessive Renal Loss

Renal excretion of potassium is determined by factors that affect the functions of the cells of the cortical connecting tubule and cortical collecting tubule. The potassium secretory functions of the principal cells in these portions of the tubule are suppressed by physiological control mechanisms during conditions of potassium depletion or hypokalemia. Therefore, daily potassium excretion will be less than 25 to 30 mmol/day when potassium concentration is in the hypokalemic range, if the controls governing potassium secretory mechanisms are operating physiologically. Quite often, however, potassium depletion is caused by inappropriately high rates of renal potassium excretion associated with dysfunctional regulation of secretory function of the distal nephron. In general, excessive urinary potassium loss leading to hypokalemia is due to mineralocorticoid excess, increased rates of tubular flow in the distal nephron, or to the presence of a nonreabsorbable anion in the tubular fluid.

**Mineralocorticoid Excess**

Aldosterone and other mineralocorticoid compounds stimulate potassium secretion by increasing the amiloride sensitive sodium conductance of the apical membrane of the principal cells, and by stimulating the activity of the sodium, potassium-ATPase located in the basolateral membrane.

*Primary hyperaldosteronism* is the uncontrolled, excessive secretion of aldosterone from a unilateral adrenal adenoma or carcinoma, or from bilateral adrenal hyperplasia. Patients frequently present with hypertension, hypokalemia, mild hypervolemia and below normal plasma renin activity.

*Cushing's syndrome* results from excessive glucocorticoid secretion from the zona fasciculata of the adrenal gland, due either to excessive stimulation by ACTH, or to adrenal carcinoma or adenoma. Although cortisol's mineralocorticoid activity is weak compared to that of aldosterone, the very high plasma levels found in Cushing's syndrome can cause potassium wasting and hypokalemia. The degree of hypokalemia is directly related to the level of cortisol secretion, the most severe in conditions with the highest hormone production. Therapeutically prescribed glucocorticoids have very weak mineralocorticoid activity and rarely produce hypokalemia.

*Congenital adrenal hyperplasia* is a syndrome characterized by excessive secretion of deoxcorticosterone (DOC) and corticosterone from the adrenal cortex due to a deficiency in 11-beta hydroxylase or 17-alpha hydroxylase, enzymes required for synthesis of cortisol. Both DOC and corticosterone possess significant mineralocorticoid effect, and therefore hypokalemia is a characteristic of this syndrome.

*Hyperreninism* can provide excessive stimulation of aldosterone leading to hypokalemia. The most common causes of sustained high renin levels are diuretic-induced hypovolemia, renal artery stenosis, malignant hypertension, and other conditions that cause persistent renal ischemia.

*Bartter's syndrome* is a rare condition in which tubular sodium loss leads to hyperplasia of the juxtaglomerular apparatus and excessive renin release that drives high rates of aldosterone secretion, leading to hypokalemia without hypertension.

*Exogenous mineralocorticoid* compounds may be ingested in licorice, chewing tobacco or snuff in sufficient quantity to occasionally cause hypokalemia. Fludrocortisone is a potent synthetic mineralocorticoid used to treat aldosterone deficiency that is capable of producing potassium depletion if taken in excess.

## Excessive Flow to the Distal Nephron

Any condition that impairs reabsorption of sodium or water in portions of the tubule proximal to the potassium secreting regions of the late distal tubule and early collecting duct can drive potassium excretion to excessive levels.

*Diuretics* that act in the ascending limb of the loop of Henle and in the proximal portions of the distal tubule are the most common examples of this (see Chapter 2).

*Metabolic acidosis* of any etiology will tend to impair proximal reabsorption of sodium and water and tend to increase distal flow rate.

*Type II renal tubular acidosis (RTA)* is characterized by reduced hydrogen ion secretion in the distal nephron and potassium and sodium depletion resulting from impaired reabsorption of sodium in the proximal tubule and accelerated potassium secretion in the distal tubule. The sodium and volume depletion stimulate the activity of the renin-angiotensin-aldosterone system so that the kaliuretic effect of the excessive distal flow rate is multiplied by greater than normal aldosterone concentration. Hypokalemia and potassium depletion are also frequent attendants of *Type I RTA*. Excessive delivery of tubular fluid to the potassium secreting portions of the nephron together with high concentrations of aldosterone provide a sustained kaliuretic drive.

**Nonreabsorbable Anions in the Distal Tubular Fluid**

If sodium ion is accompanied by a nonreabsorbable anion in the distal tubular fluid, absorption of sodium ions by the principal cells will increase the negativity of the lumen and stimulate secretion of potassium and hydrogen ions. Normally, bicarbonate ion is removed from the tubular fluid by proximal tubular reabsorption. However, in several circumstances a significant quantity bicarbonate ions enter the potassium secreting portions of the tubule, where they cannot be reabsorbed.

In *type II RTA* proximal bicarbonate reabsorption is impaired, giving rise to delivery of bicarbonate to the distal nephron along with an elevated flow of sodium and water, leading to excess potassium excretion and potentially to potassium depletion.

With *sustained vomiting*, persistent loss of hydrogen ion with the gastric contents gives rise to elevation of plasma bicarbonate concentration and filtered bicarbonate load that exceeds the reabsorption of capacity of the proximal nephron. Consequently, an elevated rate of delivery of sodium and water to the distal nephron is accompanied by nonreabsorbable bicarbonate ions. Frequently, the kaliuresis is exacerbated by a high concentration of aldosterone stimulated by the renin-angiotensin system in response to volume depletion.

*Diabetic ketoacidosis* gives rise to increased delivery of sodium and water, resulting both from glucose osmotic diuresis and metabolic acidosis. The elevated flow rate is accompanied by nonreabsorbable beta-hydroxybuturate and acetoacetate, leading to elevated rates of potassium excretion. In this case, as well as in other forms of metabolic acidosis, the kaliuresis can lead to potassium depletion with normal or even greater than normal plasma potassium concentration.

*Penicillin derivatives* are anionic compounds frequently given as sodium salts, which can stimulate potassium secretion in the distal nephron. Intravenous carbenicillin given in large dosages will promptly elevate potassium excretion.

## Gastrointestinal Loss

Loss of potassium in the feces amounts to 5 to 10 mmol/day, along with several hundred milliliters of water. However, each day 3 to 6 L of potassium-containing secretion enter the gastrointestinal lumen, most of which is reabsorbed. In patients with severe diarrhea, such as with cholera, gastrointestinal losses may be as much as 8 L per day, along with 130 mmol/day of potassium (70). Subjects with less dramatic but more prolonged diarrhea or those who chronically abuse laxatives can achieve a state of significant potassium depletion, especially if the subject consumes a diet low in potassium.

## Loss in Sweat

Hard physical work or strenuous exercise in the heat elicits elevation of body temperature and production of copious amounts of sweat. Sweating rates in excess of 1 L per hour for several hours a day are common in individuals working or participating in sports during the summer months, especially in the lower latitudes. Human sweat contains sodium and potassium in a ratio that is inversely related to aldosterone levels (71). The potassium concentration is usually between 5 and 10 mmol/L (71,72); therefore, a short bout of exercise or hard work will not endanger a person's potassium balance. However, significant potassium depletion can result from daily or frequent periods of work lasting several hours. Especially in persons eating 30 to 40 mmol/day or less, daily periods of work in high temperatures lasting a few hours will lead to a progressive depletion that may accumulate to a clinically important magnitude over a period of weeks. Rhabdomyolysis can occur after a period of intense exercise in healthy, heat acclimatized subjects who have gradually become asymptomatically potassium depleted.

Man and other terrestrial mammals have very powerful appetites for sodium, and consequently, when we work in the heat and lose sodium in sweat, we crave and seek sodium to replenish the loss. Unfortunately, we have no appetite for potassium, although we do lose significant quantities when we sweat. Before industrialization, the human diet contained approximately 200 to 400 mmol/day of potassium, and the loss of 15 to 30 mmol/day in the sweat was not of physiologic importance. Today, however, such a loss may account for half of the daily intake of potassium.

## DIAGNOSIS

The causes of hypokalemia can often be determined from the patient's history. The first consideration is the condition of the patient when the blood sample that revealed hypokalemia was drawn. If there is reason to believe that the patient's sympathetic nervous system was highly active, a transient drop in plasma potassium concentration may have resulted from a shift of potassium into the cells of the body elicited by a high level of beta adrenergic activity. Patients seen in the emergency room for treatment of trauma or severe acute illness who have a plasma potassium concentration of 3.5 mmol/L may not be potassium depleted, but may have had a redistribution of potassium following an acute elevation of beta sympathetic nervous system activity. Conversely, acidosis associated with respiratory or circulatory insufficiency, or with diabetic ketosis has the potential to shift potassium out of cells and mask potassium depletion. A more representative assessment of patients' potassium status may have to wait until a blood sample can be drawn after the level of stress and instability has subsided.

If stress and trauma are not factors, the history may reveal the cause of the hypokalemia and potassium depletion to be related to diuretic use, eating disorders, vomiting, diarrhea, laxative abuse, or low potassium, high sodium diet. When the cause can not be diagnosed from the history, additional pertinent information can be obtained from analysis of 24 hour urinary potassium excretion and the acid-base status of the patient. Hypokalemic patients with inadequate intake or extrarenal loss of potassium should excrete less than 20 to 25 mmol/day in their urine, with a urinary concentration less that 20 mmol/L; excretion rates above this may suggest some degree of impairment of renal function. In hypokalemic subjects with excessive urinary potassium loss who are also in metabolic acidosis, the underlying cause of the renal loss may be ketoacidosis, renal tubular acidosis, or salt-wasting nephropathy with renal insufficiency. In hypokalemic subjects with renal potassium wasting and metabolic alkalosis, the potassium loss may be due to a form of primary or secondary hyperaldosteronism, surreptitious vomiting or diuretic use not revealed in the history.

## TREATMENT

Treatment of hypokalemia must include efforts to correct the condition that led to potassium depletion. In addition, repletion of the deficit in total body potassium can be initiated by increasing daily potassium intake, either by enriching the potassium content of the diet and/or by taking potassium supplements. Reduction in renal potassium excretion by the use of pharmacological measures can be employed as well, to increase total body potassium balance. However, with the exception of dietary modification, all measures for treatment of potassium depletion carry some risk for development of clinically significant hyperkalemia. Therefore, it is important to consider factors that may complicate the patient's response to treatment for potassium depletion, such as reduced renal function.

## Dietary Modification

Increasing potassium intake can be accomplished by counseling from the health-care provider or a dietician; however, significant elevation of intake may not be achieved quickly. Furthermore, in addition to challenges and resistance associated with replacing preferred foods with new choices, adopting a new high potassium diet is challenging for many patients monetarily and caloricaly. Many foods rich in potassium, including fresh fruits and vegetables, dairy products and meats, are relatively expensive. And, palatable foods rich in potassium frequently also are rich in calories, which many patients are struggling to restrict. Therefore, to increase potassium intake sufficiently to correct potassium depletion through dietary modifications requires the patient to become knowledgeable not only of the potassium contents of a variety of foods, but also of the caloric contents and costs of a palatable selection of items. Certainly, dietary modifications will not work for every patient, and the prospect for success may be improved with support from a health care team that includes a professional dietician.

Interestingly, moderate restriction of sodium intake has a significant antikaliuretic impact on normal subjects and those treated with thiazide diuretics. In one study, subjects consuming a normal Western diet initially consumed 186 mmol/day of sodium and 52 mmol/day (73). They received dietary counseling for the purpose of restricting their sodium intake, and after four weeks the group's intake of sodium averaged 85 mmol/day, potassium 61 mmol/day. All subjects, those with and without diuretic treatment, experienced an increase in plasma potassium concentration of approximately 0.3 mmol/L. Even moderate reduction in sodium intake can contribute to improvement of potassium depletion.

## Correction of Magnesium Depletion

Under some circumstances potassium depletion is accompanied by magnesium depletion, particularly when the depletion of potassium results from loop diuretics, malnutrition associated with alcoholism, primary hyperaldosteronism, or from prolonged gastrointestinal loss (for review see reference 74). Some studies have shown that as many as 40% of patients with hypokalemia also present with hypomagnesemia. It has been reported that magnesium depletion exacerbates intracellular loss of potassium and makes repletion of intracellular stores more difficult. When magnesium depletion is present, potassium supplements may be less effective than expected in correcting hypokalemia. Several studies have reported greater increases in plasma potassium concentration when potassium supplements were given together with magnesium than when potassium was given alone (75). In severely potassium depleted patients, magnesium supplements, given as magnesium oxide, may be given along with potassium supplements to optimize their efficacy. At this time, definitive information concerning the relevance of magnesium depletion to repletion of potassium is not available.

## Oral Potassium Supplements

Oral supplements can be used effectively to replenish depleted potassium stores in most patients. With the formulations currently available, gastrointestinal complications rarely occur with potassium supplements, especially if supplements are taken with food. As much as 1.5 mmol/kg/day (105 mmol/day for a 70 kg man), given as either potassium chloride or potassium bicarbonate, is well tolerated in most patients. However, it may be advisable to prescribe conservatively to patients whose body mass contains a large portion of adipose tissue, i.e. BMI greater than 30. Adipose tissue has a very low potassium content and cannot take up much potassium from the extracellular space, and therefore, supplemental potassium will be excluded from distribution in much of the body mass of an obese patient. Supplements should be used with caution in patients with limited renal function or with adrenal insufficiency; close monitoring of plasma potassium concentration may be required as a precaution against development of hyperkalemia in these patients. Potassium supplements can be given safely to patients on converting enzyme inhibitors or angiotensin II receptor antagonists if renal function is normal (57), but significant hyperkalemia may develop in patients with GFR less than 50 percent of normal (76).

The magnitude of depletion can be approximated by assuming a value of 50 mmol/Kg for normal potassium content, and a value of 8% loss of total potassium content for each 1.0 mmol/L reduction in plasma potassium concentration below the normal level of 4.2 mmol/L (18,77,78). However, many circumstances commonly found in cardiovascular patients can affect the relationship between total body potassium content and plasma concentration. Therefore, any calculation of potassium deficit should be considered as only an approximation.

To achieve a rapid increase in plasma potassium concentration, oral supplements can be given in doses of 40 to 60 mmol, which will transiently raise plasma levels by 1.0 to 1.5 mmol/L (79). Only in the most severe instances of hypokalemia and potassium depletion involving the risk of ventricular arrhythmias or flaccid paralysis is intravenous potassium administration warranted, and then only to get the patient out of danger (for review see reference 61). The concentration of potassium chloride solution should be less than 60 mmol/L since higher concentrations cause a burning sensation and irritation of the vascular endothelium. Potassium should be given with saline solution, not with dextrose, which can stimulate insulin secretion and shift potassium into the cells. No more than 20 mmol/hour should be given in the absence of continuous EKG monitoring and frequent analysis of plasma potassium concentration. Once the patient is out of danger, as assessed by normalization of the EKG rather than plasma potassium concentration, potassium repletion can continue with oral administration of potassium supplements.

## Potassium Sparing Diuretics

If dietary potassium intake is adequate, potassium depletion may be treated by prescribing measures that will decrease renal potassium excretion. Potassium sparing diuretics, such as amiloride and triamterene, effectively limit potassium secretion from the principal cells of the distal nephron (see Chapter 3). The aldosterone antagonist spironolactone significantly reduces potassium excretion, especially in patients with primary or secondary hyperaldosteronism. These agents have a proven clinical record as a treatment for or preventative measure of potassium depletion associated with diuretics therapy.

# SUMMARY

Potassium depletion and hypokalemia are defined clinically as reduction in total body potassium of approximately 8%, and reduction in plasma potassium concentration from the normal value of 4.2 to 3.5 mmol/L. Under normal, steady-state conditions, plasma potassium concentration varies directly with total body potassium content, and in order for potassium in the plasma to fall from the normal level, 4.2 mmol/L, to hypokalemic levels, requires a reduction in total body potassium content of about 7 to 8% from the normal content of 3,500 mmol in a 70 kg man. Long-term depletion can result from either inadequate intake or excessive loss of potassium from the G.I. tract, the skin through sweat, or from the kidneys. Transiently, hypokalemia can follow from a shift from the extracellular compartment into the cells. Symptoms are initially vague and may be described as lack of vigor, weakness, fatigue-associated restlessness, muscular discomfort, and occasionally, exercise-induced muscle cramps. Severe potassium deficiency occurring rapidly may result in severe weakness or frank paralysis. Treatment of hypokalemia must include efforts to correct the condition that led to potassium depletion. But in addition, repletion of the deficit in total body potassium can be initiated by increasing daily potassium intake either by enriching the potassium content of the diet and/or by taking potassium supplements. Reduction in renal potassium excretion by the use of pharmacological measures can be employed as well, to increase total body potassium balance. However, with the exception of dietary modification, all measures for treatment of potassium depletion carry some risk for development of clinically significant hyperkalemia.

# SECTION II

# CARDIOVASCULAR RESPONSES TO CHANGES IN POTASSIUM

# Chapter 5

## VASCULAR CELL RESPONSES TO CHANGES IN POTASSIUM CONCENTRATION

### CELLULAR BASIS OF ATHEROSCLEROTIC LESION FORMATION

### CELLULAR BASIS OF RESTENOSIS LESION FORMATION

### REDUCTION IN PLATELET SENSITIVITY IN RESPONSE TO INCREASES IN POTASSIUM CONCENTRATION

### OXYGEN FREE RADICAL FORMATION IS INHIBITED BY ELEVATION OF POTASSIUM CONCENTRATION

### INHIBITION OF VASCULAR SMOOTH MUSCLE CELL PROLIFERATION BY ELEVATION OF POTASSIUM CONCENTRATION

### INHIBITION OF VASCULAR SMOOTH MUSCLE CELL MIGRATION BY ELEVATION OF POTASSIUM CONCENTRATION

## SUMMARY: PROPOSED MECHANISMS OF THE CARDIOVASCULAR PROTECTIVE EFFECT OF DIETARY POTASSIUM

Several laboratories have sought explanations for the apparent protective effects of diets containing high levels of potassium, beginning nearly 40 years ago. This laboratory began from the hypothesis that consuming high levels of dietary potassium results in elevation of extracellular potassium concentration, which inhibits the function of cells involved in formation of vascular lesions associated with cardiovascular diseases. The most common and clinically significant forms of vascular pathology are associated with two types of lesions: the atherosclerotic lesion and the one found in neointimal proliferative conditions that follow vascular injury. We evaluated the effects of changes in potassium concentration that could result from alterations in dietary intake on the functions of vascular cell types that give rise to these two types of lesions.

## CELLULAR BASIS OF ATHEROSCLEROTIC LESION FORMATION

Steinberg and co-workers proposed a model for the development of atherosclerotic lesions that was based on lipid infiltration and the endothelial injury hypothesis (80,81). Lesion development may be initiated by oxidation of low density lipoprotein (LDL) in the intima of the arteries where macrophages and monocytes phagocytize the oxidized LDL. If a sufficient quantity accumulates in the macrophages, they are transformed to foam cells which make up the fatty streak lesion, the first macroscopically visible element of the atherosclerotic lesion. In addition, the macrophages secrete growth factors that are mitogenic and chemotactic to smooth muscle cells. Endothelial cell injury, which may be caused by the cytotoxic effect of oxidized LDL, metabolites released from the macrophages or monocytes in the intima, or by factors in the circulation, can result in changes in endothelial cell function that contribute to the progression of the lesion. Such changes may result in adherence and penetration by monocytes as well as adherence of platelets. Platelets may then release growth-promoting factors and form aggregates with other platelets. Vascular smooth muscle cell transformation, migration and proliferation in the subintima may result from trophic factors from platelets, macrophages, endothelial cells and other cells in the developing lesion. In time, raised advanced lesions may develop. The symptoms of atherosclerosis result either from ischemia due to reduction in the lumen area by advanced lesions, or from thromboembolic events initiated by advanced lesions.

Studies in humans and animals demonstrate that one observable change within the artery prior to overt lesion formation is increased adherence of monocytes and T lymphocytes to the endothelium. These cells adhere in clusters that appear to be localized throughout the arterial tree, and many of these adherent leukocytes are attached to the endothelium at the site of flow alteration, such as at branches and bifurcations where the flow divides within various parts of the arteries. Focal cell adherence may be preceded by the deposition of lipid material beneath the endothelial cells, between the endothelium and its underlying basement membrane. The lipid material may induce the formation of specific cell-surface adhesive glycoproteins upon the surface of endothelium, which lead to binding and attachment of monocytes and T lymphocytes (80-82). The lipid material chemotactically attracts these leukocytes into the artery subjacent to the endothelium. Conversion of many of the subendothelial monocytes into macrophages or scavenger cells then takes place. These macrophages can actively bind and internalize the LDL that may be present within the intimal spaces, becoming lipid laden foam cells. Foam cell formation may lead to activation of macrophages and to genetic expression of a series of cytokines and growth-regulatory molecules. Cytokines that may be expressed by the macrophages include interleukin-1 and tumor necrosis factor-alpha, whereas T lymphocytes may express interferon gamma. The macrophages also have the capacity to express PDGF-A and -B, insulin-like growth factor-1, heparin binding EGF-like growth factor (HB-EGF), and TGF-ß1 (for review see reference 82). Many of these cytokines and growth factors are potent mitogens and chemoattractants for vascular smooth muscle cells, particularly PDGF.

Thus, a series of interactions among macrophages, T lymphocytes, overlying endothelial cells and subjacent smooth muscle cells can lead to the migration and intimal localization of macrophages and vascular smooth muscle cells that can replicate in response to the presence of growth stimulatory factors. The release of cytokines and other growth-regulatory molecules can cause expression of additional PDGF by vascular smooth muscle cells. Both PDGF and bFGF play important roles in atherosclerotic and neointimal lesion formation after balloon angioplasty. PDGF stimulates smooth muscle cell proliferation in the early stage, whereas bFGF stimulates smooth muscle cell proliferation during the chronic phase (83-88). TGF-ß1 could stimulate formation of connective tissue matrix, including collagen, proteoglycans and elastin fiber protein by smooth muscle cells within the neointima. Thus, the net results of different cellular interactions and the genetic expression in these cells could lead to a macrophage-vascular smooth muscle cell fibroproliferative response, characteristic of those observed with advanced atherosclerotic lesions.

In most circumstances, if the injury and repair were optimal, the healing events would result in a somewhat strengthened artery with no thickening of the arterial wall. But, if the injury is chronic and prolonged, as is the case with chronic hyperlipidemia, hypertension, diabetes, cigarette smoking, or combinations of these risk factors, then the injury-repair phenomenon may become excessive with time, leading to thickening of the arterial wall, to alterations within the artery that could lead to localized thrombosis, and ultimately to occlusive lesions of atherosclerosis. Thus, in all of these respects, what may begin as a protective, inflammatory response may become an excessive response that ultimately becomes a disease process.

# CELLULAR BASIS OF RESTENOSIS LESION FORMATION

Following balloon angioplasty, endothelial cell and vascular smooth muscle cell injury can produce changes in endothelial cell function that contribute to the redevelopment of a new stenotic lesion (89-92). Such changes may result in adherence and penetration by monocytes and adherence of platelets to the rough surface area of injured endothelial cells and to exposed extracellular matrix proteins in the vessel wall. Platelet adherence may then result in release of growth-promoting factors and to aggregation of other platelets. Vascular smooth muscle cell transformation, migration and proliferation in the subintima may result from trophic factors released from platelets, endothelial cells and other cells in the developing lesion. Although the pathophysiology of the process remains poorly understood, the underlying basis for restenosis is a response of the artery to vascular trauma with injury to endothelial cells and vascular smooth muscle cells. The trophic factors released in response to damage result in the exuberant growth and phenotypic conversion of the smooth muscle cells of the vascular wall. No consensus has emerged as to which specific factor(s) may be responsible for restenosis, but four interrelated processes are believed to be involved in the formation of the neointimal lesion: 1) platelet activation and aggregation, resulting in thrombosis and release of growth factors and mitogens from platelets; 2) vascular smooth muscle cell phenotypic transformation and migration from the media to intima; 3) vascular smooth muscle cell proliferation; 4) fibrosis due to the accumulation of extracellular matrix proteins.

# REDUCTION IN PLATELET SENSITIVITY IN RESPONSE TO INCREASES IN POTASSIUM CONCENTRATION

The most common causes of death in industrialized societies are myocardial infarction and stroke, usually due to thromboembolic events initiated by platelets at advanced atherosclerotic lesions. Platelet activation can be stimulated or inhibited by substances released from the endothelium or elsewhere that affect platelet function, as well as by factors activated within the platelets resulting from shear stress or surface interactions. To determine if elevations in extracellular potassium concentration directly affect platelet sensitivity to activation by external factors, an investigation was conducted using platelets obtained from freshly drawn human blood and stimulated by a range of concentrations of thrombin in buffer solution made with three different potassium concentrations, 1.9, 5.5, and 8.3 mmol/L (93). Six-point thrombin concentration response relationships were recorded. Aggregation, expressed as percent of maximum, was reduced significantly in the middle range of the concentration response relationship by elevation of potassium concentration; at the thrombin concentration of 6 U/mL, aggregation averaged 63 ± 8% in 1.9 mmol/L potassium, 50 ± 9% in 5.5 mmol/L potassium, and 41 ± 9% in 8.3 mmol/L potassium (Figure 5.1).

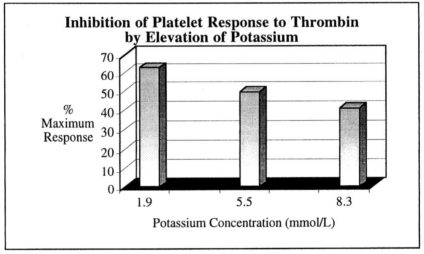

*Figure 5.1*

*Presented in the figure are aggregation responses of human platelets to thrombin in medium containing the indicated potassium concentrations. Platelet sensitivity was 50% greater in the lowest potassium concentration compared to that in the highest. From reference 93.*

Aggregation was not affected by changes in potassium concentration at either the low or the high end of the thrombin concentration curve. This 50% inhibitory effect of an increase in extracellular potassium concentration from 1.9 to 8.3 mmol/L in a relatively insensitive *in vitro* measure of platelet function offers support for a direct inhibitory action of increases in extracellular potassium concentration acting *in vivo*.

# OXYGEN FREE RADICAL FORMATION IS INHIBITED BY ELEVATION OF POTASSIUM CONCENTRATION

McCabe et al. conducted a study to determine whether physiological changes in potassium concentration affect free radical formation by vascular cells (94).

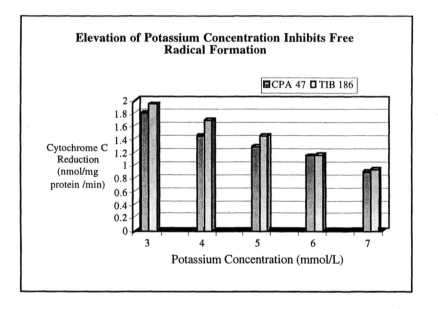

*Figure 5.2*

*Mean values of cytochrome C reduction, a measure of free-radical formation, over a 45-minute period, by endothelial cells (CPA 47) and monocyte/macrophage cells (TIB 186). Elevation of potassium concentration strongly inhibited reduction by both cell types. From reference 94.*

They assessed the effects of potassium on reactive oxygen species formation by cultured endothelial and monocyte/macrophage cells or freshly isolated human white blood cells by cytochrome c reduction or luminol chemiluminescence, respectively. Reducing potassium concentration of endothelial cell media (normally 5.1 to 6.1 mmol/l) to 3.0 mmol/L exponentially increased the rate of cytochrome c reduction, up to 8.4-fold at 2 hours; raising potassium concentration to 5.5 or 7.0 mmol/L at 1 hour reduced the maximal rate of cytochrome c reduction by 86% or 93%. Subsequent studies were done 30 to 75 minutes after media change. Extracellular potassium reduced the rate of cytochrome c reduction by 49% (CPA 47 endothelial cell line) to 55% (TIB 186 monocytes/macrophage cell line) between 3.0 and 7.0 mmol/L (Figure 5.2); the greatest decrement (20% to 26%) occurred between 3.0 and 4.0 mmol/L.

Superoxide dismutase reduced the rate of cytochrome c reduction by 62% or 50% in endothelial or monocyte/macrophage cells. Potassium had no effect on the rate of cytochrome c reduction in the presence of superoxide dismutase.

Increasing potassium concentration from 1.48 to 4.77 or 7.94 mmol/L also reduced luminol chemiluminescence in human white blood cells challenged *in vivo* by 1 to 10 mg/mL zymosan. The authors conclude that physiological increases in potassium concentration inhibit the rate of superoxide anion formation by cell lines derived from endothelium and from monocytes/macrophages, and reactive oxygen species formation by human white blood cells.

# INHIBITION OF VASCULAR SMOOTH MUSCLE CELL PROLIFERATION BY ELEVATION OF POTASSIUM CONCENTRATION

The etiologies of formation of both the atherosclerotic lesion and the neointimal proliferative lesion associated with angioplasty have been studied extensively (for review see references 80-82). Growth factors released at the site by platelets, endothelial cells, white blood cells and vascular smooth muscle cells stimulate migration of vascular smooth muscle cells from the media to the subintima, where they subsequently proliferate and synthesize extracellular matrix proteins. Migration to the point of injury is directed by platelet derived growth factor BB (PDGF-BB) (83), while basic fibroblast growth factor (bFGF) and PDGF-BB are the prominent regulators of vascular smooth muscle cell proliferation (86-88). Transforming growth factor beta 1 (TGF-ß1) stimulates synthesis of collagen and other extracellular matrix proteins by vascular smooth muscle cells in the subintima (88).

Recently, we analyzed the effects of changes in extracellular potassium concentration in a physiological range on the actions of PDGF-BB, bFGF and 5% fetal bovine serum (5% FBS) to stimulate proliferation of vascular smooth muscle cells *in vitro* (95). The responses of cells derived from explants of pig coronary arteries to the cytokines most important in the etiology of vascular lesions were assessed in media with potassium concentrations ranging from 3 to 6 mmol/L. Both DNA synthesis and cell proliferation were analyzed during changes in potassium concentration lasting from one to seven days. The effect of potassium concentration on vascular smooth muscle cell proliferation stimulated by PDGF-BB (20 ng/mL) is presented in Figures 5.3.

A significant inverse relationship was found between extracellular potassium concentration and vascular smooth muscle cell proliferation stimulated by either PDGF-BB, bFGF or 5% FBS. Proliferation stimulated by 20 ng/ml PDGF-BB ranged from 143 ± 21% in potassium concentration of 3 mmol/L to 58 ± 7% in potassium concentration of 6 mmol/L (100% = value in potassium concentration of 4 mmol/L).

The limits of proliferation stimulated by bFGF were 114 ± 39% in potassium concentration of 3 mmol/L and 84 ± 29% in potassium concentration of 6 mmol/L, while the range of proliferation stimulated by 5% FBS was from 106 ± 10% in potassium concentration of 3 mmol/L to 77 ± 4% in potassium concentration of 6 mmol/L.

A significant inverse relationship also was found between potassium concentration and thymidine incorporation in vascular smooth muscle cells stimulated by 20 ng/ml PDGF-BB. Raising potassium concentration to 6 mmol/L reduced $^3$H-thymidine to 61 ± 4% of the value observed in the control potassium concentration (4 mmol/L).

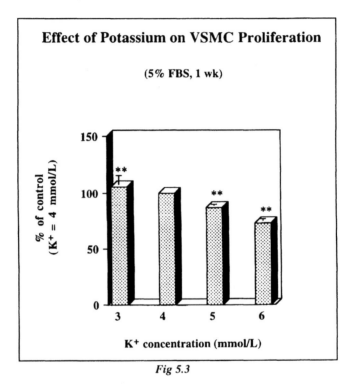

*Fig 5.3*

*Elevation of potassium concentration in the medium inhibited proliferation of vascular smooth muscle cells. Values are expressed as % of control, the value measured at medium concentration of 4.0 mmol/L. From reference 95.*

Similarly, DNA synthesis stimulated by bFGF (25 ng/mL in DMEM) was inhibited by increases in potassium concentration. $^3$H-thymidine incorporation ranged from 106 ± 6% in potassium concentration of 3 mmol/L to 76 ± 5% in potassium concentration of 6 mmol/L. Thus, physiological elevation of potassium concentration opposes the effect of PDGF-BB, bFGF and serum cytokines to stimulate DNA synthesis and proliferation.

PDGF-BB and bFGF were chosen for study because of their documented importance in formation of vascular lesions associated with atherosclerosis and balloon injury. At potassium concentrations from 3 to 6 mmol/L, cell counts in medium containing PDGF-BB ranged in a nearly linear manner from 135% of the control value in 3 mmol/L potassium to 63% in a potassium concentration of 6 mmol/L. Cell proliferation stimulated by bFGF was also sensitive to increases in potassium concentration, although the magnitude of the inhibition was approximately half as great as in the studies done with PDGF-BB. Thymidine incorporation showed highly significant inverse relationships to medium potassium concentration with both PDGF-BB and bFGF as agonists. Serum was also used as an agonist because it contains other cytokines in addition of PDGF and bFGF that may contribute to the proliferative response of vascular smooth muscle cells. The inhibitory effect of increases in potassium concentration against 5% FBS were quantitatively similar to those observed with PDGF and bFGF. Therefore, the inhibitory action may be effective against generalized mechanisms regulating proliferation.

The effects of increases in potassium concentration on cell proliferation and DNA synthesis may be mediated by stimulation of the activity and/or expression of sodium, potassium-ATPase in the cell membrane, which would decrease intracellular sodium concentration and increase the concentration gradient driving the sodium-calcium exchange mechanism. This is the hypothesis proposed by Canadry et al. to account for the inhibition by potassium of cell proliferation and DNA synthesis in glial cells in culture (96). In studies in vascular smooth muscle cells, the reduction in tension associated with elevation of potassium concentration in the physiologic range has been attributed by Haddy and co-workers to an increase in sodium, potassium-ATPase activity (97,98). Also, Songu-Mize, Caldwell and Baer demonstrated that physiologic increases in dietary potassium intake or in plasma potassium concentration act *in vivo* to increase vascular smooth muscle sodium, potassium-ATPase activity (99). Intracellular sodium concentration is known to increase markedly prior to initiation of vascular smooth muscle proliferation (100); increases in extracellular potassium concentration from 3 to 7 mmol/L were shown by McCabe and Young (101) to reduce by 74% the increase in intracellular sodium concentration in vascular smooth muscle just prior to serum-stimulated proliferation. Jones recorded an increase sodium efflux in response to elevation of extracellular potassium concentration from vascular smooth muscle cells *in vitro* (102). Similarly, in other cell types increased expression of sodium, potassium-ATPase in the cell membrane has been associated with reduction in intracellular sodium concentration (103).

Any reduction in intracellular sodium concentration associated with elevation of extracellular potassium concentration could be expected to stimulate calcium extrusion from the cell by the sodium-calcium exchange mechanism, and subsequently, lead to a reduction in intracellular calcium concentration. The multiple signaling pathways activated by growth factors (both G-protein linked and tyrosine kinase linked) invariably include increases in intracellular calcium (104,105). Any increase in calcium extrusion, resulting from increased activity of the sodium, potassium-ATPase or sodium-calcium exchange, would down-regulate the calcium-dependent signaling pathways leading to proliferation.

Elevation of extracellular potassium concentration within the physiological range was found to inhibit *in vitro* vascular smooth muscle cell thymidine incorporation and proliferation stimulated by PDGF-BB, bFGF and 5% FBS. Suppression of these functions could be responsible in part for the reduction in formation of atherosclerotic and neointimal proliferative lesions observed in animals given high potassium diets.

# INHIBITION OF VASCULAR SMOOTH MUSCLE CELL MIGRATION BY ELEVATION OF POTASSIUM CONCENTRATION

The etiology of the neointimal proliferative lesion that follows angioplasty has been studied extensively by others, and is known to include several alterations in the function of cells of the arterial wall (90-92). Of significant importance are migration from the media to the subintima and subsequent proliferation of medial vascular smooth muscle cells. During migration to the intima, the cells change from the differentiated, contractile phenotype to the dedifferentiated, synthetic state that is associated with proliferation. Platelet derived growth factor (PDGF) is a potent chemoattractant and mitogen for cells of mesenchymal origin, and for vascular smooth muscle cells.

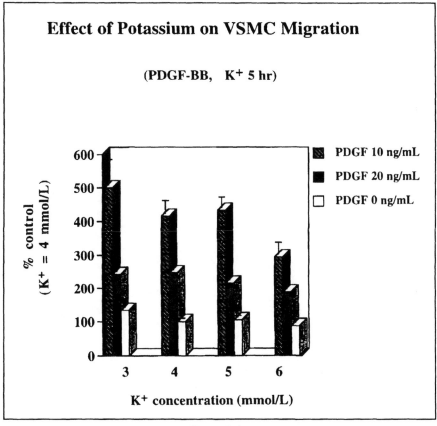

**Figure 5.4**

*Cells were exposed to PDGF-BB and/or to changed medium potassium concentration for five hours. Data are presented as percentages; 100% is the mean value for migration in potassium concentration of 4.0 mmol/L and 0 ng/mL PDGF-BB within each experiment. Elevating potassium concentration inhibited migration with and without PDGF stimulation. From reference 106.*

Recently, we tested the hypothesis that elevation of extracellular potassium concentration inhibits vascular smooth muscle cell migration (106). An *in vitro* design utilizing a modified Boyden chamber was used so that precise control of potassium concentration and other variables could be maintained. In a short-term study, vascular smooth muscle cells exposed to no growth factors and to a control potassium concentration of 4.0 mmol/L migrated through the membrane to the lower chamber, reaching a mean count of 93 ± 10 cells in the five hour experiment. Data from the experiment in which the cells were exposed to PDGF-BB and/or to changed medium potassium concentration for five hours are presented in Figure 5.4, expressed as percentages; 100% is the mean value for migration in potassium concentration of 4.0 mmol/L and 0 ng/mL PDGF-BB within each experiment. The stimulatory effect of PDGF-BB on migration has been shown by others to decline with increases in concentration above 10 ng/mL (83), and the same trend was observed in this study as well, with the group mean of the 10 ng/mL counts being significantly greater than the 20 ng/mL group mean at each level of potassium concentration.

With increasing potassium concentration, migration was significantly inhibited ($p < 0.02$, two-way ANOVA; for 10 ng/mL, $r = -0.22$, $p < 0.01$; for 20 ng/mL, $r = -0.13$, $p < 0.09$). In the wells with 10 ng/mL PDGF-BB, the migration values ranged from 500 ± 86% for 3.0 mmol/L potassium to 294 ± 44% in the wells containing 6.0 mmol/L potassium concentration ($p < 0.03$).

The effects of long-term exposure of the cells to selected extracellular potassium concentrations were also investigated. Cells were grown in medium with concentrations of 3.0, 4.0, 5.0 or 6.0 mmol/L for three to four weeks prior to being added to the wells of the Boyden chamber. In the upper and lower chambers, the potassium concentrations were the same as those in which the cells had been grown. Migration was assessed with either no PDGF-BB or 20 ng/mL in the lower chambers. The migration data expressed as percentage of the control values are presented in Figure 5.5.

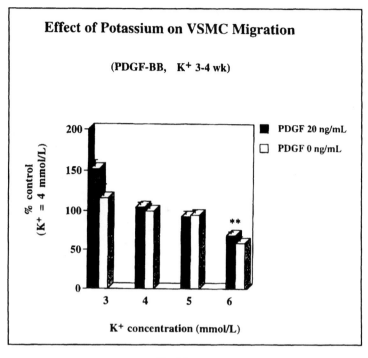

*Fig 5.5*

*Presented here are data from migration experiments using cells grown for three to four weeks in medium containing the potassium concentrations indicated. Migration was inhibited in the wells containing cells grown in higher potassium concentrations. From reference 106.*

The effects of increases in potassium concentration on cell migration may be mediated by stimulation of the activity and/or expression of sodium, potassium-ATPase in the cell membrane, which would decrease intracellular sodium concentration and increase the concentration gradient driving the sodium-calcium exchange mechanism. And since cellular locomotion required for migration is mediated by coordinated, calcium-dependent changes in the polymerization and depolymerization of actin-containing microfilaments (107), any reduction in intracellular calcium activity associated with elevation of extracellular potassium concentration could be expected to reduce migration.

Migration of vascular smooth muscle cells into the subintima is an early and quantitatively important step in atherosclerotic and restenosis lesion formation. In the rat, most of the cells of the injury lesion following angioplasty are progeny of cells that migrated from the media, while in the swine and human restenosis lesions, the modified smooth muscle cells that comprise the lesion are derived from cells that originated in the intima as well as those from the media (92)

## SUMMARY:     PROPOSED MECHANISMS OF THE CARDIOVASCULAR PROTECTIVE EFFECT OF DIETARY POTASSIUM

On the bases of the results of the studies reviewed above, and the work of others concerning the general mechanisms involved in vascular lesion formation, we propose that high levels of potassium in the diet can inhibit the following mechanisms that could account for potassium's cardiovascular protective effects:

> *platelet aggregation and thrombus formation*
> *free radical formation and LDL oxidation*
> *vascular smooth muscle cell proliferation*
> *vascular smooth muscle cell migration*

From this series of studies, it is clear that elevation of extracellular potassium concentration, even in the physiological range, can significantly influence functions of the cells of the vascular system. These effects may provide protection against cardiovascular diseases that are related to lipid peroxidation, foam cell formation and accumulation in the subintima of arteries, migration and proliferation of vascular smooth muscle cells in the subintima, and thrombus and embolus formation.

# Chapter 6

# INHIBITION OF THROMBOSIS AND STROKE BY ELEVATION OF POTASSIUM

### INHIBITION OF EXPERIMENTAL CORONARY AND CAROTID ARTERY THROMBOSIS BY ELEVATION OF POTASSIUM CONCENTRATION

### PROTECTION AGAINST STROKE IN THE STROKE-PRONE RAT MODEL BY HIGH DIETARY POTASSIUM INTAKE

### EVIDENCE FROM POPULATION BASED STUDIES OF PROTECTION AGAINST STROKE BY HIGH DIETARY POTASSIUM INTAKE

### SUMMARY

# INHIBITION OF EXPERIMENTAL CORONARY AND CAROTID ARTERY THROMBOSIS BY ELEVATION OF POTASSIUM CONCENTRATION.

The most common causes of death in industrialized societies are those resulting from coronary or cerebral artery occlusion by thromboembolic events initiated by platelets at advanced atherosclerotic lesions. Platelet activation can be stimulated or inhibited by substances released from the endothelium or elsewhere that affect platelet function, as well as by factors activated within the platelets resulting from shear stress or surface interactions. As discussed in the previous chapter, elevation of potassium concentration reduces the sensitivity of platelets for a number of agonists (93). To determine if the *in vitro* findings were also valid *in vivo*, we studied the effect of elevation of potassium concentration on thrombus formation in a well-studied experimental animal model.

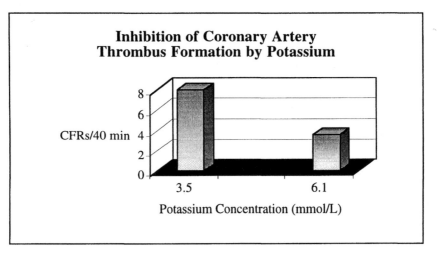

*Figure 6.1*

*Elevation of plasma potassium concentration from 3.5 to 6.1 mmol/L reduced the rate of cyclical blood flow reductions (CFRs) in the coronary arteries of dogs more than 50% from 8.0 to 3.7 per 40 minute observation period. From reference 93.*

In the model developed by Folts, the endothelium of the vessel was damaged by external compression of the artery after which a critical stenosis was produced at the damaged section with a Plexiglas occluder (108). If the artery is prepared properly a repeating pattern of cyclical flow reductions (CFR's) continues in a consistent manner for several hours. During this time the effect of interventions on the rate of CFR's could be used to assess the efficacy of their antithrombotic actions. An acute increase in the potassium concentration in this model drastically reduced the rate of CFR's (93) (Figure 6.1). In a group of 10 dogs intravenous potassium infusion increased the concentration from $3.53 \pm 0.05$ to $6.10 \pm 0.09$ mmol/L, which resulted in a reduction in the rate of CFR's from $8.0 \pm 0.6$ to $3.7 \pm 1.0$ ($p < 0.01$) during the 40 minute KCl infusion.

We also analyzed the effects of acute increases of potassium concentration on the thrombogenic effects of epinephrine. Intravenous infusion of epinephrine increased the rate of CFR's more than 60%, from $7.1 \pm 0.5$ to $11.5 \pm 0.7$ in the 40 minute period following infusion. However, as a result of raising plasma potassium to approximately 6 mmol/L while epinephrine was continuously administered, the frequency of CFR's was significantly reduced from $11.5 \pm 0.7$ to $7.7 \pm 1.1$ ($p < .01$) in the 40 minute period. Potassium infusion with elevation of plasma concentration was capable of opposing completely the thrombogenic effect of epinephrine infusion. This dramatic reduction in rate of thrombus formation was observed in the same model used by others to establish the antithrombotic efficacy of aspirin and other interventions subsequently shown to be clinically effective.

A similar preparation was used to induce a pattern of cyclical flow reductions in the carotid artery of rabbits. In 4 of the 5 rabbits used, increasing potassium concentration from approximately 3.5 to 5.5 mmol/L completely inhibited thrombus formation and reduced the rate of cyclical flow reductions to zero. Results from one of these rabbit experiments are illustrated in Figure 6.2. In this case the potassium concentration before KCl infusion was 3.54 mmol/L. In less than 5 minutes after the start of potassium infusion thrombus formation at the site of endothelial damage and constriction was completely inhibited. At that time plasma potassium concentration had risen to 5.07 mmol/L.

For the duration of the experiment during which thrombus formation was totally inhibited, plasma potassium concentration varied from 5.61 to 4.83 mmol/L, demonstrating that acute changes in potassium concentration of < 1.5 mmol/L may be highly effective in inhibiting thrombus formation in stenosed vessels with damaged endothelium. This *in vivo* finding may be closely relevant to a mechanism explaining the protective effect of potassium-rich diets against stroke in humans and animals.

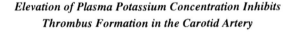

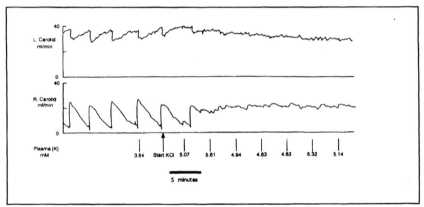

**Figure 6.2**

*Shown here are blood flow data from the left and right carotid arteries of an anesthetized rabbit whose right carotid artery had been prepared with a section of damaged endothelium and a partial constriction placed over the damaged section. This preparation results in periodic formation of thrombi at the point of damage. The progression of thrombus development can be monitored from the blood flow through the artery. When the vessel is completely occluded, the thrombus can be dislodged by gentle mechanical agitation after which blood flow returns to the initial level. A new thrombus will begin to develop after the previous one is dislodged, giving rise to a cyclic pattern of blood flow reduction, as shown in the initial portion of the tracing for the right carotid. The left carotid shows compensatory increases in flow, out of phase with the decreases in the contralateral vessel. When plasma potassium concentration was increased by iv infusion, thrombus formation was abolished. From reference 13.*

# PROTECTION AGAINST STROKE IN THE STROKE-PRONE RAT MODEL BY HIGH DIETARY POTASSIUM INTAKE

A spontaneously hypertensive rat that is prone to develop stroke has been studied extensively in many labs throughout the world. When the rats are fed a diet containing 4% sodium chloride for 17 weeks, mortality, principally from strokes, is more than 80%. Most are thromboembolic infarctions, although many are the result of hemorrhage from cerebral arteries.

Tobian and co-workers conducted an extensive series of investigations of the effect of increasing potassium content of the diet on stroke mortality in this strain of rats (109). In one study they compared mortality rates in two groups of rats fed the 4% sodium chloride diet (110). In the untreated group, with a dietary potassium of 0.75%, mortality rate was 83% after 17 weeks, while in a second group, with a dietary percentage of 2.1% potassium chloride, only one of the 50 rats died at the end of the 17 week study, yielding a 2% mortality rate. The blood pressure of the potassium supplemented group was significantly less than the control group's, which was a partial explanation for the protective effect of the potassium supplements. However, the investigators selected subgroups having equivalent blood pressures, with a mean of 212 mmHg for the control and the potassium supplemented group. In this comparison in which blood pressure was not a factor, and which is presented graphically in Figure 6.3, there was a 9% mortality rate in the potassium treated group and a 64% mortality rate in the untreated group.

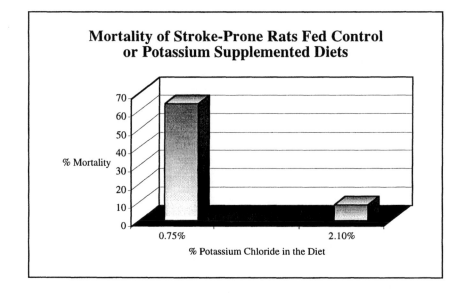

***Figure 6.3***
*Mortality of two groups of stroke-prone spontaneously hypertensive rats with matched mean arterial pressures. Mortality was greatly reduced in the group fed the high potassium diet. From reference 110.*

These findings from the main study and analysis of the subgroups indicates that elevation of dietary potassium intake protects against stroke in this model indirectly by reducing blood pressure and by mechanisms independent of the level of arterial pressure.

In a second study of the same model, rats were fed the same two diets for 22 weeks (111). In the control group with the 0.75% dietary potassium intake, there was a 64% mortality rate, while in the group receiving 2.11% potassium, there was a 6% mortality rate. The brains of all the survivors were examined for the presence of hemorrhages. In the survivors of the control group, 40% showed evidence of a previous cerebral hemorrhage, while none of the 34 survivors in the high potassium group had any sign of hemorrhage. In a similar study saggital sections of the brain were made at 0.5 mm intervals and examined for the presence of brain infarcts. Among the surviving animals on the normal diet, 36% showed evidence of brain infarction, however in the animals given the 2.11% potassium diet, incidence of infarction was only 2%.

The investigators also studied stroke prone rats given the normal and the high potassium diet for eight weeks, before there was any mortality. The brains were examined for evidence of hemorrhage, and in the normal potassium intake group the incidence was 36% vs. 6% in the group that received the high potassium diet.

This extensive series of investigations revealed the existence of a mechanism associated with high dietary intake of potassium that is strongly protective against stroke. However, the nature of the mechanism cannot be assessed from the results, nor can it be determined if the mechanism is operable in other strains of rats or in other species.

# EVIDENCE FROM POPULATION BASED STUDIES OF PROTECTION AGAINST STROKE BY HIGH DIETARY POTASSIUM INTAKE

The potential protective effect of potassium against strokes has been studied using the perspective of epidemiological studies in population groups. One of the earlier and more influential studies was conducted by Khaw and Barrett-Connor in a population based cohort of 859 men and women aged 50 to 79 years in Southern California (112). They tested the hypothesis that a high dietary intake of potassium may be related to a lower risk of stroke in this population. The cohort was drawn from a geographically defined upper-middle-class white community. Dietary intake was obtained from 24 hour recall of food intake. After 12 years of follow-up, 24 stroke-associated deaths had occurred. The relative risks of stroke-associated mortality in the lowest tertile of potassium as compared to that in the top 2 tertiles combined, were 2.6 (p = 0.16) in men and 4.8 (p = 0.01) in women. The lowest tertile of intake was less than 59 mmol/day, the middle level was 59 to 76 mmol/day, and the highest tertile was intake greater than 76 mmol/day. In multivariate analyses, a 10 mmol/day increase in intake was associated with a 40% reduction in the risk of stroke associated mortality (p < 0.001). The effect of potassium was independent of other dietary variables and of known cardiovascular risk factors.

The relationship between reported dietary potassium intake and incidence of stroke and stroke related mortality was assessed in the Honolulu Heart Study, which included 7,591 Japanese men living in Hawaii (113). Daily potassium intake quintiles were established, with the low intake group having an intake of less than 1,469 mg/per day (37 mmol/day) and the highest group reporting greater than 2,776 mg (71 mmol) per day. During the 16 years of follow-up, 408 cases of stroke were identified; among the 33 fatal strokes, there was a significant inverse relationship between intake and incidence rate (p < 0.002). The associations between intake and incidence of non-fatal thromboembolic strokes and hemorrhagic strokes were not significant.

Sasaki and co-workers, using World Health Organization statistics, analyzed the relationship between potassium intake and other dietary variables with the gender and age-specific stroke mortality rates for the period between 1986 and 1988 (114). Stroke mortality rates and 24 hour urinary excretion data from 58 surveyed populations from 17 countries described in 24 published articles were analyzed by Pearson correlation and multiple regression analysis. Significant inverse correlations were observed between urinary potassium excretion and stroke mortality for all age groups of men and women, with the exception of the oldest class of women (from 65 to 74 years). Significant correlations were also recorded between urinary sodium excretion, urinary sodium/potassium ratio, intake of saturated fat and alcohol consumption, and stroke mortality. The range of dietary potassium excretion means was from 42.8 mmol/24 hour from Japan to 72.5 mmol/24 hour for Australia.

Data from the Health Professionals Follow-Up Study, which began in 1986, were analyzed by Ascherio et al. to address the hypothesis that high potassium intake reduces the risk of stroke in U.S. men (115). 43,738 eligible men, 40 to 75 years old, without diagnosed cardiovascular diseases or diabetes, completed a semi-qualitative food frequency questionnaire in

1986, and were then followed for eight additional years. 328 strokes, 210 ischemia, 70 hemorrhagic, and 48 unspecified, were documented. The multivariate relative risk of stroke of any type for men in the top fifth of potassium intake (median intake of 110 mmol per day) versus those in the lowest fifth whose median intake was 61 mmol per day was 0.62 (p = 0. 007) (Figure 6.4). The results for ischemic stroke were similar, although there was no reduction in risk for hemorrhagic stroke. The inverse association between potassium intake and risk of stroke was stronger in hypertensive than normal men, and was not altered by adjustment for blood pressure levels.

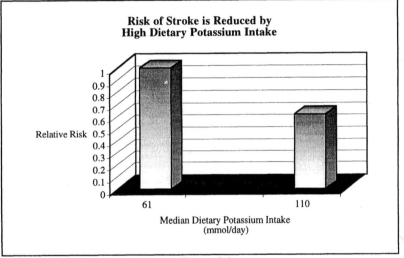

***Figure 6.4***

*Relative risk of stroke was 0 .62 in the quintile with the highest median potassium intake compared to that of the lowest potassium quintile. From reference 115.*

Subsequently, the same group investigated the relationship between intake of potassium and other anions on the incidence of stroke among U.S. women followed prospectively for 14 years in the Nurses' Health Study (116). 85,746 women aged 34 to 59 years, free of diagnosed cardiovascular disease and cancer, completed dietary questionnaires that were used to calculate intakes of potassium and other cations. 690 incidents of stroke were recorded, including 129 subarachnoid hemorrhages, 74 intraparenchymal hemorrhages, 386 ischemic strokes, and 101 strokes of undetermined type. Intakes of potassium, calcium, and magnesium were each inversely associated with age and smoking-adjusted relative risks of ischemic stroke. The median potassium intake for the lowest quintile was 52 mmol per day, and for highest quintile the median intake was 91 mmol per day; relative risk for ischemic stroke for the highest quintile was 0.66 (p = 0.03) compared to the lowest quintile. Adjustments for other cardiovascular risks, including history of hypertension, attenuated the associations; in the multivariate analysis, women in the highest quintile of potassium intake had a relative risk of ischemic stroke of 0.72 (p for trend = 0.10).

Recently, the clinical relevance of hypokalemia associated with a low-dose diuretics was assessed using data from the Systolic Hypertension in the Elderly Program, in which 4,126 elderly hypertensive participants were randomized to low dose chlorthalidone or placebo (117). After one year of treatment, 7.2% of participants randomly assigned to active treatment had serum potassium less than 3.5 mmol/L compared to 1% of participants randomized to placebo. During the subsequent four years, 177 participants experienced stroke, 215 experienced coronary events, and 323 died. Within the active treatment group the risk of stroke was 72% lower among those who had normal serum potassium levels compared to those who experienced hypokalemia (p < 0.05). After adjustment for known risk factors and study drug dose, the participants who received active treatment and who experienced hypokalemia had a similar risk of cardiovascular events, coronary events and stroke as those randomized to placebo. Several decades of clinical experience have proven the effectiveness of low dose chlorthalidone in reducing cardiovascular risk, and yet, based on these data from the SHEP study, the increase in risk associated with moderate hypokalemia is great enough to offset those well-established benefits of chlorthalidone.

The association of dietary potassium intake with stroke mortality in a general population was examined among the participants in the first National Health and Nutrition Examination Survey (NHANES I) (118). Dietary potassium intake determined by 24 hour dietary recall at baseline, during the period from 1971 to 1975, was available for 9,866 subjects, and follow-up continued through 1992. Mean age and dietary potassium at baseline were 55 years and 53 mmol per day. African-Americans reported significantly lower potassium intake than whites (41 vs 56 mmol per day). 304 stroke deaths were reported. For men, stratified by tertile of dietary potassium intake, age-adjusted stroke mortality rates per 1000 person-years for the lowest dietary potassium groups were significantly higher than for the highest intake group, for both white (1.94 vs 1.17; relative risk, 1.66; 95% confidence interval, 1.3 - 2.14) and African-Americans and (5.08 vs 1.19; relative risk, 4.27; 95% confidence interval, 1.88 - 9.19).

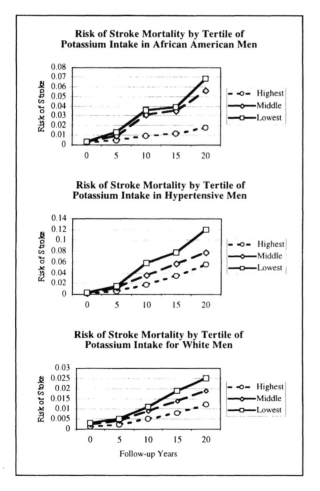

*Figure 6.5*

*Risk of stroke mortality by tertile of potassium intake in African-American men (top), hypertensive men (middle), and white men (bottom), controlled for caloric intake, body mass index, age, smoking and serum cholesterol.*

For women, there was no significant difference in stroke mortality between similar levels of potassium intake for either white or African-Americans.

After stratification by hypertensive status, stroke fatality rates were significantly different by tertile of dietary potassium only for hypertensive men. There was no stroke mortality difference by potassium intake in hypertensive women or non-hypertensive men and women. Multivariate analysis, which included control for caloric intake and other baseline cardiovascular risk factors, revealed that only in African-American men and hypertensive men was lower dietary potassium intake a significant predictor of stroke mortality. For African-American men, those with the lowest potassium intake (< 32 mmol per day), compared with those with the highest potassium intake (>56 mmol per day), had a 167% higher stroke mortality. For hypertensive men, those with the lowest potassium intake (< 45 mmol per day) had an 88% higher stroke mortality rate compared with those with potassium intake greater than 66 mmol per day (Figure 6.5).

## SUMMARY

Collectively, these studies, most of which have been published recently, present convincing support for an inverse relationship between dietary potassium intake and risk of stroke. None of the individual studies presents evidence linking potassium intake to stroke risk for all members of the population; however, there is information from several of the studies indicating that stroke risk in hypertensive individuals is inversely related to dietary intake or plasma potassium concentration. It is also noteworthy that a strong protective effect of high potassium intake was measured in African-American men, the segment of the population that has the highest stroke risk.

Each of the studies makes valuable contributions to our understanding of potassium and the risk of stroke. However, each is inadequate in a crucial aspect of design that undoubtedly limits the information that can be derived from the studies: each analyzed the relationship of risk to an insufficiently broad range of potassium intakes. In most of the studies, the lowest tertile or quintile of potassium intake analyzed was close to the national average U.S. potassium intake, 50 to 60 mmol/day. Only in the African-American group analysis in the NHANES I study was the lowest intake group within a range comparable to the intake rates of tens of millions of inhabitants of industrialized cultures who live on potassium-poor diets. And even in that group, the upper limit of intake, 32 mmol/day, is approximately the average intake, not the lowest intake, recorded in several studies of African Americans living in the stroke belt the southeast United States. Furthermore, in that analysis stroke rate of the low group was compared to that of the highest intake group, whose lower limit was only 56 mmol/day. Therefore, in addition to what this group of studies has already demonstrated, their results also suggest that if the relationship between a wider range of potassium intakes and risk of stroke were analyzed, even more convincing evidence for a protective effect of potassium would emerge.

# Chapter 7

# INHIBITION BY POTASSIUM OF ARTERIOSCLEROSIS AND ATHEROSCLEROTIC LESION FORMATION

## ETIOLOGY OF LESION FORMATION

## POTENTIAL MECHANISMS OF PROTECTION AGAINST LESION DEVELOPMENT BY ELEVATION OF POTASSIUM CONCENTRATION

## INHIBITION BY DIETARY POTASSIUM OF CORONARY ARTERIOSCLEROTIC LESION FORMATION IN A RABBIT MODEL

## EVIDENCE FROM POPULATION BASED STUDIES OF PROTECTION BY POTASSIUM AGAINST DEVELOPMENT OF ARTERIOSCLEROTIC DISEASE

## SUMMARY

## ETIOLOGY OF LESION FORMATION

The cellular mechanisms responsible for atherosclerotic lesion formation
were discussed in detail in Chapter 5. In the general case, the formation of
the lesions is believed to begin with infiltration of low density lipoproteins
(LDL) into the subintima, oxidation of the LDL by reactive oxygen species
(ROS) from monocytes, macrophages, endothelial cells and vascular smooth
muscle cells, recruitment of large numbers of additional monocytes to the
subintima by chemotactic properties of oxidized LDL and cytokines formed
in response to oxidized LDL, phagocytosis of the modified LDL by
macrophages and their subsequent conversion to foam cells, and secretion of
growth factors mitogenic to smooth muscle cells. Accumulation of the foam
cells results in fatty streak formation, which is the characteristic of the early
vascular lesion. The possibly rate-limiting step in lesion development is the
oxidation of LDL in the intima of arteries by reactive oxygen species (ROS).
The oxidized LDL and cytokines released from the macrophages initiate
responses in the overlying endothelial cells, leading to platelet adherence
and activation resulting in secretion of trophic substances that stimulate
migration and hyperplasia of the vascular smooth muscle cells in the
subintimal layer. In time, raised advanced lesions may develop. The
symptoms of atherosclerosis result either from ischemia due to reduction in
the lumen area by advanced lesions, or from thromboembolic events
initiated by advanced lesions.

## POTENTIAL MECHANISMS OF PROTECTION AGAINST LESION DEVELOPMENT BY ELEVATION OF POTASSIUM CONCENTRATION

On the bases of the results of the studies reviewed in Chapter 5, and the
work of others concerning the general mechanisms involved in vascular
lesion formation, we propose that high levels of potassium in the diet can
inhibit the following mechanisms that could account for potassium's
cardiovascular protective effects:

> *platelet aggregation and thrombus formation*
> *free radical formation and LDL oxidation*
> *vascular smooth muscle cell proliferation*
> *vascular smooth muscle cell migration*

These effects may provide protection against cardiovascular diseases that are related to lipid peroxidation, foam cell formation and accumulation in the subintima of arteries, migration and proliferation of vascular smooth muscle cells in the subintima, and thrombus and embolus formation.

## INHIBITION BY DIETARY POTASSIUM OF ARTERIOSCLEROTIC LESION FORMATION IN A RABBIT MODEL

To determine whether or not changes in dietary potassium intake could affect the severity of arteriosclerotic lesion development *in vivo*, the cholesterol fed rabbit model was studied (119). Two groups of rabbits were fed diets containing 2% cholesterol and either a low potassium content, 0.4%, or a normal potassium percentage, 1.5%. The feed-in period lasted 6 weeks. The rabbits were sacrificed, and the hearts were removed for analysis of the arteries.

Lesions in small and medium sized arteries and arterioles were observed in the myocardium from both groups of cholesterol fed rabbits. Small arteries and primary and secondary arterioles showed both subintimal focal micronodular and intraluminal deposits along with diffuse subintimal linear deposition of homogenous (mildly oxyphilic) hyaloid material confined within the circumferential limits of the internal elastic membrane. The subintima of the affected arteries showed abundant accumulation of foam cells, which in some smaller arteries resulted in greater than 90% reduction in lumen diameter. In some of the larger arterioles, there was mild medial muscular hypertrophy. These are similar to those seen in the early stages of coronary artery disease in man.

Plasma potassium concentration in the normal dietary potassium intake group averaged 4.27 ± 0.67 mmol/L and in the low dietary potassium intake group the mean was 3.90 ± 0.34 mmol/L. Plasma cholesterol, HDL, LDL, triglycerides and body weight gain values from the two groups were similar. The percentage of abnormal vessels, those showing foam cells in the intima, present in the myocardia of the animals from the two groups are presented graphically in Figure 7.1. The percentage of abnormal arteries in the normal potassium intake group averaged 4.2 ± 0.4%, while in the low potassium intake group the mean was 6.4 ± 0.5%, 51% more than the normal dietary potassium intake group (p < 0.01).

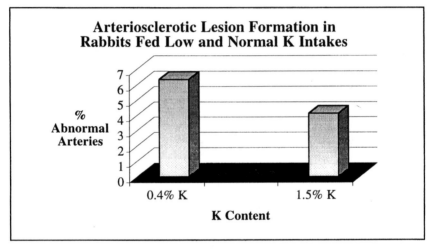

***Figure 7.1***
*Rabbits fed a diet with low potassium content, 0.4%, had 6.4% of coronary arteries that showed signs of arteriosclerotic lesion formation, 51% more than rabbits eating diet with normal potassium content, 4.2%. From reference 119.*

Vascular lesions associated with hypercholesterolemia are initiated by phagocytosis of oxidatively modified LDL cholesterol by macrophages in the subintima, between the endothelial cells of the intima and the smooth muscle of the media. With continued accumulation of LDL in the macrophages, they become filled with lipid material, assuming the morphology of the foam cell. In large arteries focal masses of foam cells may be visible as fatty streak lesions at developing atherosclerotic plaques. In small vessels the presence of subintimal foam cells is a characteristic of early development of arteriosclerosis. In this study, possibly because the high cholesterol feeding period was limited to six weeks, we failed to observe atherosclerotic plaque formation in the large coronary arteries. The type of lesion we observed is of interest in that it is similar to that seen in human myocardial resistance arteries early in the course of arteriosclerotic disease.

The mechanism of the effect of potassium intake on formation of this type lesion may be associated with the inverse relationship between potassium concentration and oxygen free radical formation we observed in a previously completed study (94). Elevation of potassium concentration of the medium from 3.0 to 7.0 mmol/L reduced the rate of free radical formation (measured as reduction of cytochrome C) 55% from the monocyte/macrophage cell line, TIB 186. The greatest effect of potassium concentration was between 3.0 and 4.0 mmol/L, where a 26% reduction was measured. An increase in free radical formation associated with a reduction in ECF potassium concentration may have increased the rate of oxidative modification of LDL cholesterol, thereby exacerbating foam cell formation as observed in the tissue from the low potassium intake group. From these results, we conclude that long-term, moderately low dietary potassium intake may exacerbate development of foam cell lesions in the small arteries of the myocardium, possibly due to an elevation of free radical formation and LDL oxidative modification associated with reduced potassium intake.

# EVIDENCE FROM POPULATION BASED STUDIES OF A PROTECTIVE EFFECT OF POTASSIUM AGAINST ATHEROSCLEROTIC VASCULAR DISEASE

At this time, no population-based studies designed to test the hypothesis that potassium can protect against atherosclerotic vascular disease have been completed. However, some information concerning potassium's protective effect can be derived from studies of primitive tribes that eat diets containing very high amounts of potassium and very low amounts of sodium. At least 14 of these tribes from nearly every continent have been studied during the last 50 years; observations were made concerning dietary content of sodium and potassium and other nutrients, blood pressure level, incidence of hypertension, heart failure, stroke, and apparent coronary artery disease (1,2,120-132). The names and origins of these groups are presented in Table 7.1.

*Table 7.1*

*Populations eating primitive diets that have low incidence of cardiovascular diseases*

*Aita people, Solomon Islands (120)*
*Australian aborigines (2)*
*Botswana natives (121)*
*Carajas Indians, Brazil (122)*
*Cuna Indians, Panama (123)*
*Eskimos, Greenland (124)*
*Kenya natives (125)*
*Melanesian, northern Cook Islands (126)*
*New Guinea natives (127)*
*South African natives (128)*
*Tarahumara Indians, northern Mexico (1,129)*
*Ugandan natives (130)*
*West China natives (131)*
*Yanomamo Indians, Brazil (132)*

In all groups that have been studied, no more than 1% of the people have high blood pressure, and the level blood pressure does not increase with age, even in the 5 to 10% of the populations that live into their 60's or 70's. Not only do these aboriginal groups have almost no hypertension, but they also rarely have strokes, coronary artery disease or other ailments related to atherosclerotic vascular disease. Certainly these observations do not establish a definitive link between high potassium intake and protection against cardiovascular diseases; other factors common to these cultures may be responsible for the reduced incidence of atherosclerotic disease, such as, low sodium intake, low caloric intake, high fiber intake, or low protein intake. These studies were not designed to provide proof of the relationship between one factor and risk of cardiovascular disease; however, the observations are at least consistent with the hypothesis that potassium provides cardiovascular protection.

Additional indirect support concerning the potential protective effect of potassium comes from analyses of the risk of cardiovascular disease in vegetarian populations living within industrialized Western cultures. In studies in vegetarians in Boston (133), monks in Holland and Belgium (134), Seventh Day Adventists in Australian (135), and vegetarians in Tel Aviv (136), incidences of hypertension, strokes and coronary artery disease are very low, nearly as low as in the primitive population groups, discussed above. Likewise, the blood pressure of the vegetarian groups does not rise with age as it does in non-vegetarian populations. Plasma potassium concentration of the subjects in these studies was not measured, and only in the Tel Aviv study was urinary electrolyte excretion analyzed; the potassium to sodium ratio in the urine of the vegetarians was 1.41 while in the non-vegetarians it was 1.04. The vegetarian diets consumed in all of these studies undoubtedly have higher potassium contents than the customary Western diet, and this higher potassium content may have contributed to the apparent protection against cardiovascular diseases.

The putative atherosclerotic protective effect of potassium receives more direct support from a recent analysis of data from the Systolic Hypertension in the Elderly Program (SHEP), a five-year randomized, placebo-controlled clinical trial of chlorthalidone-based treatment of isolated systolic hypertension in older persons (117). After one year of treatment, 7.2% of the participants randomized to active treatment had serum potassium concentration less than 3.5 mmol/L, compared with of 1% of the participants randomized to placebo. During the four years after the first annual visit, 451 participants experienced a cardiovascular event, including 215 coronary events and 177 strokes. The participants who received active treatment and who experienced hypokalemia had a similar risk of cardiovascular events, coronary events, and stroke as those randomized to placebo. Within the active treatment group, the risk of these events was 51%, 55%, and 72% lower, respectively, among those who had normal serum potassium levels compared with those who experienced hypokalemia ($p < 0.05$) (Figure 7.2). There were no significant differences between the two groups' blood pressure, serum creatinine, glucose, cholesterol, or HDL-cholesterol; however, serum triglycerides and uric acid levels were higher in the hypokalemic group than in the normal potassium group. Thus, the participants who had hypokalemia after one year of treatment with a low-dose diuretic did not experience a reduction in cardiovascular events achieved among those who did not have hypokalemia. Most of the cardiovascular events were directly related to atherosclerotic disease, and the very strong reduction in risk associated with normal potassium concentration versus potassium concentration below 3.5 mmol/L represents the most significant evidence available so far supporting potassium's ability to protect against atherosclerotic events.

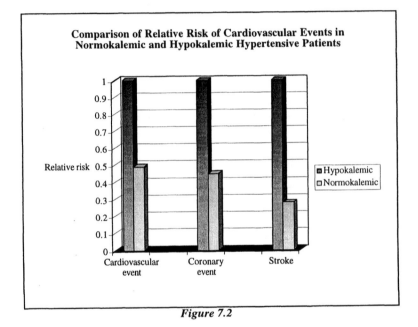

**Figure 7.2**

*Risk of all cardiovascular events was much greater in hypokalemic than in normokalemic patients treated with diuretics for hypertension. From reference 117.*

## SUMMARY

The laboratory studies described in previous chapters suggest that small elevations of extracellular potassium concentration can affect the cells of the vascular system in ways that could provide protection against development of atherosclerosis and other cardiovascular diseases. The affected mechanisms include: 1) platelet aggregation, 2) free radical formation from monocytes, macrophages and other cells, 3) vascular smooth muscle cell migration, and 4) vascular smooth muscle proliferation. In the one laboratory study conducted specifically to determine if alteration of potassium concentration resulting from dietary modification could affect development of vascular lesions, we found that reduction in intake significantly increased the occurrence of coronary artery lesions characterized by foam cell formation, lesions similar to early arteriosclerosis in human coronary artery disease. No investigations in man have tested specifically for a similar relationship, but inferences can be made from studies of cardiovascular disease incidence such as the SHEP study in which potassium concentration was measured and found to be inversely related to occurrence of cardiovascular events that are caused by atherosclerotic vascular disease. Additionally, scores of studies of incidence of cardiovascular disease in primitive populations and in sub-populations within Western cultures have reported the coincidence of low rates of cardiovascular disease and high potassium intake in the diet.

While these observations do not establish a definitive link between high potassium intake and protection against cardiovascular diseases in man, the observations are at least consistent with the hypothesis that potassium provides cardiovascular protection.

# Chapter 8

# NEOINTIMAL PROLIFERATION AND RESTENOSIS FOLLOWING ANGIOPLASTY ARE INHIBITED BY DIETARY POTASSIUM SUPPLEMENTATION IN EXPERIMENTAL MODELS

### ETIOLOGY OF RESTENOSIS

### INHIBITION OF NEOINTIMAL LESION FORMATION FOLLOWING ANGIOPLASTY IN ANIMAL MODELS BY ELEVATION OF DIETARY POTASSIUM INTAKE

### SUMMARY

## ETIOLOGY OF RESTENOSIS

Percutaneous transluminal coronary angioplasty has been used extensively since the technique was introduced 20 years ago by Gruntzig (137). Treatment of stable and unstable angina, and acute myocardial infarction are the most common application of the procedure, accounting for more 350,000 cases each year. Currently, in addition to the original procedure involving inflation of a balloon at the site of the lesion, other approaches are also employed, including atherectomy, laser ablation, and endovascular stenting. However, with all of these interventions, the benefits are short-lived in many patients due to redevelopment of stenoses at the site of the initial lesion.

A reduction in lumen area may result either from growth of the vessel wall into the lumen, or from remodeling of the same amount of wall material within a vessel of smaller overall cross-sectional area around a smaller lumen. In man following angioplasty, restenosis results principally from development of a neointimal proliferative lesion with growth of the wall into the lumen. Endothelial cell and vascular smooth muscle cell injury can produce changes in endothelial cell function that contribute to the redevelopment of new stenotic lesion. Such changes may result in adherence and penetration by monocytes and adherence of platelets to the rough surface area of injured endothelial cells and to exposed extracellular matrix proteins in the vessel wall (89-91). Platelet adherence may then result in release of growth-promoting factors and to aggregation of other platelets. Vascular smooth muscle cell transformation, migration and proliferation in the subintima may result from trophic factors released from platelets, endothelial cells and other cells in the developing lesion (92,138). Although the pathophysiology of the process remains poorly understood, the underlying basis for restenosis is a response of the artery to vascular trauma with injury to endothelial cells and vascular smooth muscle cells. The trophic factors released in response to damage result in the exuberant growth and phenotypic conversion of the smooth muscle cells of the vascular wall. Four interrelated processes are believed to be involved:

1)      thrombosis, due to laceration of the original plaque and exposure of its interior to blood;

2)      vascular smooth muscle cell migration from the media to intima;

3)      vascular smooth muscle cell proliferation;

4)      fibrosis due to the accumulation of extracellular matrix proteins.

Because our previously described experience showing that elevation of potassium concentration inhibited the function of the cells involved in neointimal proliferation, we analyzed the response to changes in dietary potassium intake of neointimal proliferation after angioplastic balloon injury in two experimental animal models.

# INHIBITION OF NEOINTIMAL LESION FORMATION FOLLOWING ANGIOPLASTY IN ANIMAL MODELS BY ELEVATION OF DIETARY POTASSIUM INTAKE

## Studies in the Rat Carotid Artery Model of Balloon Injury

The rat model of balloon injury in the carotid artery was used to assess potassium's effect on neointimal proliferation (139). Three groups of Sprague Dawley rats weighing 250-340 g were used. For 14 days prior to surgery they were fed specially formulated diets, containing either 0.1% potassium for the low intake group, 1.5% for the normal intake group, or 4.0% for the group eating the high potassium intake. One half of the potassium was added as KCl and half as $KHCO_3$. All had a sodium content of 0.24%. Standard rat laboratory diets produced by Teklad/Harlan have potassium contents of approximately 1.0%.

After the 14 days of modified diet, the rats were anesthetized and the right carotid artery was exposed via a midline incision. The vessel was isolated, including the initial portion of the external carotid. A 2F Fogarty balloon embolectomy catheter was introduced into the right external carotid and passed caudally to the aorta. The balloon was inflated and withdrawn approximately 30 mm cephalically, then deflated and advanced back into the aorta. The procedure was repeated six times, after which the catheter was removed and the external carotid ligated. Care was taken so as to not compromise flow through the internal carotid artery.

Following surgery, the animals consumed the modified diets for an additional 14 days at which time the carotid arteries were removed, fixed and mounted in paraffin, sectioned and stained with hematoxylin and eosin

(H&E) for histologic analysis. There were 25, 19, and 26 animals analyzed in the low, normal and high intake groups, respectively.

Group mean plasma potassium concentration of blood drawn from the indwelling catheters was significant affected by dietary potassium content; group mean and standard errors were 4.26 ± 0.12 mmol/L for the low intake group, 5.22 ± 0.19 mmol/L for the normal group, and 5.80 ± 0.23 mmol/L for high intake group. The potassium concentration of the group eating standard lab diet averaged 4.98 ± 0.12 mmol/L. Plasma renin activity (PRA) was measured in some animals in each group; group mean values were 5.4 ± 0.9, 3.6 ± .5, and 2.1 ± 0.3 ng AI/ml/hr for the low, normal and high groups, respectively. Mean arterial pressure of the rats was unaffected by the range of potassium in the diets. The group means were 96 ± 2 mmHg for the low intake group, 99 ± 2 mmHg for the normal, and 101 ± 3 mmHg for high intake group. The group eating standard lab chow averaged 98 ± 2 mmHg.

Sections of normal carotid artery had an intact layer of endothelial cells, a media containing elastin fibers and a normal adventia. In balloon injured artery sections from the low and normal intake groups, there was extensive neointima development. The neointima comprised smooth muscle cells with abundant extracellular matrix. In the normal intake group, the character of the neointima was similar to that of the animals in the low intake group. The neointimal response in the high potassium intake group was significantly attenuated compared to that of the other groups.

A consistent, significant inverse relationship was observed between the level of potassium intake and the neointimal to medial area ratio (Figure 8.1). The group mean values for the ratio of neointimal area to medial area for the low, normal and high intake groups were, 0.447 ± 0.106, 0.384 ± 0.116, and 0.240 ± 0.046, respectively. The 47% reduction in the proliferation index associated with only dietary modification of potassium strongly supports the potential protective actions of potassium on the vascular response to balloon injury.

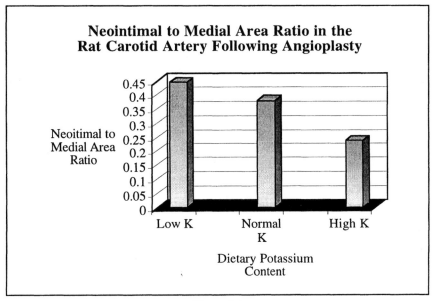

*Figure 8.1*

*Presented here is an index of neointimal proliferation, the neointimal to medial area ratio, of groups of rats fed low, normal and high potassium containing diets following carotid artery balloon angioplasty. From reference 139.*

## Studies in the Swine Coronary Artery Balloon Injury Model

The lesion that develops in this model is similar in many respects to that found following angioplasty in the human coronary artery (90-92). Because we observed in the rat study that elevation of potassium intake from normal to higher than normal was associated with the greatest reduction in lesion formation, we chose dietary intake levels in the present study (140) of normal and eight-fold greater than normal. The animals were fed the experimental diets beginning 14 days before angioplasty and continuing 14 days after the procedure, when the animals were sacrificed.

Two groups of 7 castrated male swine were included in the study. The diets were prepared to our specifications by Purina Test Diets (Richmond, IN). The two preparations were identical except for the potassium content. The "normal" diet contained 0.25% potassium (from native ingredients) and the high potassium diet had a content of 2.0% (additional potassium was added as KCl). Both contained 0.25% sodium. The animals consumed 3% of their body weight per day of the diet and gained weight normally on both diets.

Both groups were fed their prescribed diets for 14 days prior to the angioplasty procedure. On the day of the procedure, they were intubated and a surgical level of anesthesia was maintained with halothane and oxygen. Under aseptic conditions the right femoral artery was exposed and cannulated with an 8 or 9 F sheath. The swine received 200 U/kg of heparin given intravenously. Coronary balloon angioplasty was performed on an unbranched section of the proximal left circumflex artery, with six inflations, each for 30 seconds, to give a diameter approximately 25% to 30% greater than the diameter of the vessel. Throughout the procedure the animals' blood pressure, heart rate and ECG were monitored continuously. After the procedure, the femoral artery was ligated and the wound was closed.

The animals were maintained on the specified diets for an additional 14 days. The experiment was terminated on the 14th day after angioplasty when the animals were anesthetized, the chest was opened and the heart was removed for gross and histologic examination of the injured vessels. Histological sections were coded and examined blindly as to the treatment of the animal. The presence of medial dissection, any disruption of internal or external elastic lamina, and the amount of thrombotic material were quanitated using a modification of the scoring system described by Karas et al. (141). Briefly, the degrees of medial laceration and external elastic lamina stretch were given a grade of 0 for no injury, 1 for partial medial laceration, 2 for complete medial laceration, and 3 for complete medial laceration and stretching of the external elastic lamina. The amount of thrombotic material at the injury site was evaluated using a scoring system of 0-5, with zero indicating no thrombotic material discernible within the neointima and 5 indicating a well formed thrombus within the injured vessel segment. Digital images of two to three histologic vessel cross sections from uninjured segments proximal and distal to the injured vessel segment were used to obtain the mean values for: vessel outer diameter, vessel wall area, lumen area and vessel wall thickness. The maximal neointimal thickness was also measured in the injured segment using the digital image and computer software. These values from the uninjured and injured vessel segments were used to calculate the mean neointimal area of the injured segment by subtracting the mean vessel wall area of the uninjured segment (containing only media) from the mean vessel wall area of the injured segment (containing both media and neointima).

The fluorscopically estimated vessel diameter prior to angioplasty averaged 2.4 ± 0.2 mm in the normal K group, and 2.4 ± 0.1 mm in the group eating the high potassium diet. The inflated diameter of the balloons used in the normal potassium group average 3.1 ± 0.2 mm, and in the high potassium group the mean value was 3.0 ± 0.1 mm. Vessel dimensions at the lesion site 14 days after angioplasty are given in Table 8.1.

*Table 8.1*
**Vessel Dimensions at the Lesion Site**

|  | Outer diameter mm | Wall area mm$^2$ | Medial area mm$^2$ | Neointimal area mm$^2$ | Lumen Area mm$^2$ | Wall/ Lumen ratio |
|---|---|---|---|---|---|---|
| **Normal K** |  |  |  |  |  |  |
| mean | 3.91 | 3.66 | 2.92 | 0.74 | 3.05 | 1.96 |
| Std error | 0.11 | 0.37 | 0.28 | 0.10 | 0.12 | 0.25 |
|  |  |  |  |  |  |  |
| **High K** |  |  |  |  |  |  |
| mean | 2.74 | 2.76 | 2.43 | 0.33 | 3.36 | 1.25 |
| Std error | 0.07 | 0.07 | 0.08 | 0.04 | 0.07 | 0.03 |
|  |  |  |  |  |  |  |
| P < | n.s. | 0.034 | n.s | 0.004 | 0.039 | 0.027 |

Although the outer diameters of the two groups were similar, the lumen area of the high intake group averaged 3.36 ± 0.07 mm$^2$, significantly larger than the area of the group on normal K intake, 3.05 ± 0.12 mm$^2$. The wall area to lumen area ratio of the high intake group was significantly less than that of the normal intake group, 1.25 ± 0.03 vs 1.96 ± 0.25.

After 14 days of feeding, blood samples were collected from the femoral artery under anesthesia at the time of the angioplasty procedure. The normal K group mean value was $3.07 \pm 0.19$ mmol/L while the mean from the high K group was $3.95 \pm 0.12$ mmol/L, significantly greater than the normal K group mean ($p < 0.003$). At the time of sacrifice a second sample was collected by direct puncture of the aorta. The mean values were not significantly different for the two groups; the normal K mean was $3.64 \pm 0.14$ mmol/L and the high potassium group mean was $4.09 \pm 0.26$ mmol/L ($p < 0.191$).

Oversize balloon injury in the normal swine coronary artery produced damage to the media, which in most cases resulted in laceration. In many of the vessel segments evaluated, the media was completely transected in one location and the external elastic lamina had been stretched. The injury scores for the two groups were similar, $2.53 \pm 0.06$ for the normal group, and $2.59 \pm 0.16$ in the high potassium group. This level of injury indicates that in the majority of the specimens, the media were partially or completely lacerated. At 14 days after angioplasty, the discontinuity of the media was filled by neointima. The neointima consisted of primarily smooth muscle cells that had a fusiform to somewhat stellate morphology with pale eosinophillic cytoplasm, consistent with the secretory, proliferative smooth muscle phenotype. An abundant extracellular matrix material surrounded the smooth muscle cells. There were occasional small blood vessels deep within the neointima and occasional inflammatory cells, primarily macrophages and a few lymphocytes. Deep within the neointima and along the edge of the external elastic membrane there was often an accumulation of thrombotic material. The presence of thrombotic material was more frequent and more severe in specimens from the normal potassium group than in the high potassium group.

The neointimal thickness (Figure 8.2) in the hyperkalemic group averaged 58% less than that of the normal K group ($267 \pm 18$ μm vs $708 \pm 111$ μm, $p < 0.002$); the neointimal area (Figure 8.3) was also markedly less in the high potassium group than in the normal K group, $0.33 \pm 0.04$ mm$^2$ vs $0.74 \pm 0.10$ mm$^2$ ($p < 0.004$).

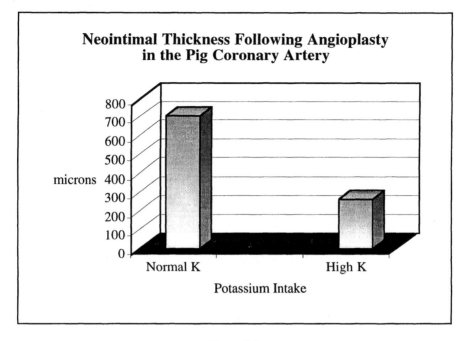

**Figure 8.2**
*Neointimal thickness was significantly less in the group fed the high potassium diet than in the normal diet group. From reference 140.*

Neointimal area to total wall area ratios were computed (Figure 8.4); in the normal potassium group the ratio averaged 0.199 ± 0.018, significantly greater than the ratio computed for the elevated potassium group, 0.120 ± 0.015 (p < 0.006). Similarly, the neointimal to medial area ratio was significantly less in the high potassium group than in the low intake group, 0.138 ± 0.19 vs 0.252 ± 0.28, respectively.

The thrombus score data are presented in Figure 8.5. The high K group's score averaged 72% less than the score from the normal K group, 0.59 ± 0.20 vs 2.14 ± 0.20 (p < .006).

We demonstrated previously that elevation of extracellular potassium concentration markedly reduced the rate of two processes believed to be causally related to neointimal proliferation and restenosis lesion development: thrombus formation and proliferation of vascular smooth muscle cells. Potassium's potential effectiveness in inhibiting thrombosis was analyzed using an *in vivo* model in the dog circumflex (Chapter 6).

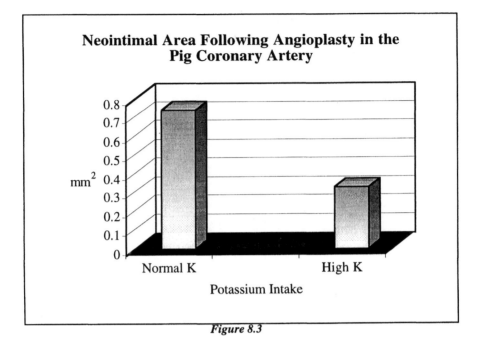

*Figure 8.3*

*Neointimal areas was significantly less in the group fed the high potassium diet than in the normal diet group. From reference 140.*

An acute increase in the potassium concentration from $3.53 \pm 0.05$ to $6.10 \pm 0.09$ mmol/L reduced by 56% the rate thrombus formation. The importance of thrombus formation in neointimal development was emphasized by the experiment by Willerson et al. (142) who observed a strong correlation between frequency of cyclical blood flow reductions in damaged coronary arteries of dogs and the severity of neointimal thickening over a 21 day period. When inhibitors of thrombus formation were given to the animals, well-correlated reductions in cyclical blood flow reductions and neointimal thickening were recorded. In the present study the finding of a thrombus score in the high potassium group 72% lower than in the normal intake group of swine is consistent with an antithrombogenic effect of potassium being causally related to the reduction in neointimal proliferation observed in the high potassium intake group. We also analyzed potassium's effect on proliferation of vascular smooth muscle cells *in vitro* (95,101). As described in a preceding chapter (Chapter 5), vascular smooth muscle cells were exposed to medium with final potassium concentrations ranging in 1 mmol/L increments from 3 to 7 mmol/L.

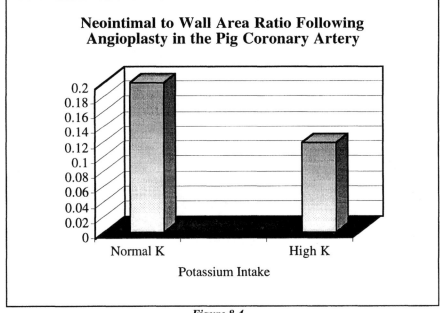

**Figure 8.4**

*Neointimal to total wall area ratio was less in the high K intake group than in the control group. From reference 140.*

Increasing potassium concentration for 7 days from 3 to 7 mmol/L reduced the cell proliferation rate by 61%, while raising the concentration from 3 to 4 mmol/L reduced the rate by 18%. An effect of elevated extracellular potassium concentration associated with greater than normal intake on either vascular smooth muscle cell proliferation or thrombus formation could provide the mechanism for the observed inverse relationship between potassium intake and neointimal lesion formation.

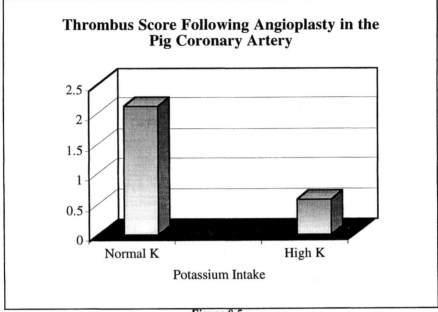

**Figure 8.5**

*Thrombus scores were reduced more than four-fold in the high intake group. From reference 140.*

## SUMMARY

The observation of potassium's effectiveness to markedly reduce neointimal development in the rat carotid artery and swine circumflex artery following angioplasty are consistent with our previous findings of potential vascular protective effects in *in vitro* experiments (94,95,101,106), during short-term *in vivo* experiments in dogs (93), and in long-term studies in rabbits (119). The mechanisms of potassium's effects may include inhibition of thrombus formation and a direct inhibitory effect on proliferation of vascular smooth muscle cells. This series of positive results in a wide range of models and time courses provides strong support for the long-term protective actions of elevation of potassium intake.

# Chapter 9

# EVIDENCE OF AN INVERSE RELATIONSHIP BETWEEN DIETARY POTASSIUM INTAKE AND BLOOD PRESSURE

## BLOOD PRESSURE REGULATION AND THE ETIOLOGY OF HYPERTENSION

## CHANGES IN BLOOD PRESSURE CONTROL FUNCTIONS OF THE KIDNEY ASSOCIATED WITH CHANGES IN POTASSIUM INTAKE AND PLASMA POTASSIUM CONCENTRATION

## REDUCTION IN BLOOD PRESSURE BY ELEVATION OF POTASSIUM INTAKE IN EXPERIMENTAL HYPERTENSION

## REDUCTION IN BLOOD PRESSURE IN HYPERTENSIVE PATIENTS BY POTASSIUM SUPPLEMENTATION

## BLOOD PRESSURE REDUCTION BY ELEVATION OF POTASSIUM INTAKE AND OTHER DIETARY MODIFICATIONS -- THE *DASH* TRIAL

# EPIDEMIOLOGICAL EVIDENCE THAT HIGH DIETARY POTASSIUM INTAKE PROTECTS AGAINST HYPERTENSION

## SUMMARY

## BLOOD PRESSURE REGULATION AND THE ETIOLOGY OF HYPERTENSION

Blood pressure is regulated by a control system that also regulates body fluid balance (for review, see references 143-146). The system operates in such a way that when arterial pressure increases, the output of fluid by the kidneys also increases, so that for each rate of daily intake of fluid there must be exactly the same rate of daily fluid output. Furthermore, the rate of renal excretion of fluid is very strongly affected by the level of arterial pressure perfusing the kidney; very small increases in renal perfusion pressure stimulate large increases in renal excretion of sodium and water. On the other hand, the level of arterial pressure is a function of the amount of fluid retained in the body; as total body fluid volume increases, blood volume and cardiac output also increase, resulting in an elevation of arterial pressure. An equilibrium is established at which a sufficient amount of fluid is retained in the body to provide a level of arterial pressure that will promote a rate of renal excretion of fluid that will exactly match the rate of fluid intake into the body. This kidney-fluid balance-blood volume-blood pressure negative feedback control system is highly effective in maintaining arterial pressure at a constant level, as long as the intake of sodium and water remain unchanged and the intrinsic function of the system is not altered. When the system is functioning normally, urinary excretion can rise several hundred percent in response to steady-state increases in arterial pressure of only a few mmHg; therefore, even a very large increases in fluid intake will not cause significant hypertension, as long as the intrinsic function of the control system is not impaired.

Sustained hypertension will result if the ability of the kidneys to increase their rate of fluid excretion in response to an elevation in renal perfusion pressure is impaired. When this occurs, a positive fluid balance will develop at the normal level of arterial pressure, creating an elevation of extracellular fluid volume and blood volume. The positive balance thereby will give rise to an elevation of arterial pressure. Fluid retention will continue and renal perfusion pressure will rise progressively until it reaches the level at which renal excretion matches the level of intake. This new equilibrium will again be characterized by a balance between intake and excretion of fluid, but the steady-state level of arterial pressure will be elevated above normal. Patients with essential hypertension have apparently normal renal excretion of fluid and electrolytes, and they are in daily fluid balance. However, they have greater than normal arterial and renal perfusion pressure, and it is the high level of perfusion pressure that maintains renal fluid and electrolyte excretion at a rate that is in balance with intake.

The changes in renal function that can result in sustained hypertension can be described and classified in three categories, presented in Table 9.1:

*Table 9.1*

***Three Categories of Changes in Renal Function That Can Cause Hypertension***

---

*1. Increased preglomerular vascular resistance, resulting from:*
>   A. *arteriosclerotic, atherosclerotic or congenital constriction*
>      *of renal arteries*
>   B. *afferent arteriolar constriction due to nephrosclerosis,*
>      *sympathetic stimulation, or high levels of circulating*
>      *vasoconstrictors*

*2. Decreased glomerular filtration capacity resulting from:*
>   A. *glomerular inflammation*
>   B. *thickening or damage of the glomerular membrane*
>   C. *increased plasma colloid osmotic pressure.*

*3.   Increased tubular reabsorption of sodium and water due to*
*greater than normal concentrations of:*
>   A. *aldosterone*
>   B. *angiotensin II*
>   C. *other antinatriuretic substances.*

---

As a group, patients with essential hypertension have reduced renal blood flow even in the early course of the condition, and the reduction becomes more severe with time as the hypertension progresses (for review, see reference 144). The changes in the renal vasculature are even more strikingly apparent when the elevation in renal vascular resistance is considered; even in the early stages of the disease renal resistance may be increased as much as 100%. Glomerular filtration rate early in the disease may not be decreased, probably because perfusion pressure is greater than normal, although later in the progression, GFR falls and filtration fraction increases. In some varieties of essentials hypertension, aldosterone and angiotensin II concentrations may be greater than normal, and their antinatriuretic actions contribute to the alteration in renal function that gives rise to hypertension.

# ALTERATIONS IN BLOOD PRESSURE CONTROL FUNCTIONS OF THE KIDNEY ASSOCIATED WITH CHANGES IN POTASSIUM INTAKE AND PLASMA POTASSIUM CONCENTRATION

Increases in extracellular potassium within the physiological range affect several process these that may alter renal function. First, the rate of activity of sodium, potassium-ATPase in vascular smooth muscle is increased by elevation potassium concentration within the physiological range (97,99,103), and this activation is linked to an increased rate of calcium extrusion from the cells carried by the sodium-calcium exchange mechanism. These mechanisms are involved in the vasodilation seen in most vascular beds including the kidney in response to physiological increases in potassium concentration (97,98). Second, the mechanism regulating the renin release may also be affected by hyperkalemia's effect on membrane potential and intracellular calcium concentration (46). Finally, sodium and chloride reabsorption proximal to macula densa may be inhibited by elevation of potassium concentration, either in the proximal tubule or in the thick ascending limb of Henle's loop (147-150).

## GFR, Renal Blood Flow, and Renal Vascular Resistance

Previous investigations have provided inconsistent evidence that increases in potassium concentration altered renal function in ways that are related to the blood pressure control functions described above. Renal vasodilation in response to hyperkalemia has been reported by some (151,152) but not all groups studying the subject (153,154); hyperkalemia has been similarly associated with stimulation (155,156), inhibition (154,157), and no effect (153) on renin release or plasma renin activity in a variety of preparations. The discrepancies are probably the result of the use of different concentrations of potassium in the various experiments; up to certain potassium concentrations in the high physiological range, increases produced no change or a reduction in intracellular calcium activity in vascular smooth muscle. In several species, reductions in renal resistance have been reported in response to elevation of plasma potassium concentration up to approximately 6 mmol/L (151,152). However, above this level further increases in potassium are associated with membrane depolarization (158,159). The results reporting renal vasoconstriction in response to intraarterial infusion of potassium chloride probably are due to local elevation of potassium concentration well above 6 mmol/L.

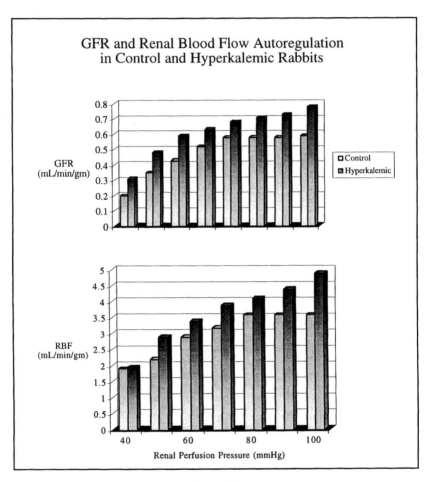

**Figure 9.1**

*Presented here are GFR (top) and renal blood flow rate (bottom) responses in anesthetized rabbits during controlled reductions in renal perfusion pressure. The hyperkalemic group that received KCl infusion i.v. had poor autoregulatory efficiency, but much lower vascular resistance at all levels of perfusion pressure. From reference 156.*

Recently, we conducted experiments designed to clarify the relationship between changes in potassium concentration within the physiological range and regulation of renal hemodynamics. The autoregulatory capabilities of the renal vascular bed was studied in anesthetized dogs (155) and rabbits (156) during controlled step reductions in renal perfusion pressure in normal groups and in groups whose potassium concentration was elevated within the physiological range by intravenous infusion of potassium chloride. The ranges of potassium concentration studied were from 3.2 to 6.8 mmol/L in rabbits, and from 3.5 to 5.7 mmol/L in dogs. In both species the increase in potassium concentrations resulted in profound increases in renal blood flow and GFR. In the dog experiments renal blood flow was elevated by 45% and GFR by 35% at the 120 mmHg perfusion pressure level. Autoregulation of both GFR and renal blood flow were severely impaired by the increase in potassium concentration in both groups. Renal blood flow and GFR data from the study using rabbits are presented in Figure 9.1. Notice the severe impairment of autoregulatory ability, particularly of GFR.

The elevation of GFR resulting from the increase in potassium concentration is noteworthy since not all renal vasodilators increase filtration rate; for example, acetylcholine and papaverine both increase renal flow by approximately 100% while decreasing filtration rate by as much as 60% (160). Increases in GFR associated with vasodilators may be attributed to a greater impact on afferent arteriolar tone than on efferent tone. This particular effect of potassium on the renal vasculature may be especially beneficial to hypertensive patients who increase their dietary potassium intake.

The effect on regulation of renal hemodynamics did not wane over the time-course of the studies. If the effects persist over periods of days and weeks, these renal mechanisms could alter the relationship between arterial pressure/renal perfusion pressure and the rate of sodium excretion.

## Sodium Reabsorption

Acute elevation of plasma potassium concentration produces a prompt and prominent diuresis and natriuresis, as shown by Addison in 1928 (161). In addition to the hemodynamics effects, elevation of potassium concentration has been reported to have direct effects on tubular transport of sodium. Brandis et al. presented evidence that increases in potassium concentration in the plasma inhibit proximal tubular sodium reabsorption, a 1.0 mmol/L increase in potassium producing a 68% reduction in sodium reabsorption (147). The mechanism may be attributed to a progressive decrease in plasma bicarbonate concentration, which may accompany potassium chloride infusion. More recently, several studies have observed a prominent inhibitory effect on sodium and chloride transport in the loop of Henle (148-150). In this case, the mechanism of inhibition seems to be associated with an increase in intracellular potassium concentration resulting in a reduction in electrochemical potential gradient favoring absorption of sodium and potassium by the sodium, potassium, two chloride cotransport in the thick a ascending limb.

Earlier, we had shown that a natriuresis of modest proportions occurs on the first day of potassium loading in intact dogs, and in adrenalectomized dogs maintained of fixed aldosterone replacement; in the animals without feedback control of aldosterone, an increase of 217% of control sodium excretion occurred on the first day following potassium loading (Figure 9.2) (47,162). The natriuresis continued for three days before the animals returned to balance. The cumulative negative balance was 84 mmol in this group of 20 kg dogs that did not have functional feedback control of aldosterone; that amount was equal to approximately three times the daily rate of sodium intake. This experiment revealed the natriuretic effect of a small increase in plasma potassium concentration, 0.8 mmol/L, that is frequently obscured by the antinatriuretic influence of a rise in aldosterone concentration resulting from the elevation in potassium.

Effects such as these that increase the rate of sodium excretion at a given level of perfusion pressure have the potential to reduce steady-state arterial pressure. Therefore, an effect of potassium on the pressure-natriuresis mechanism may be responsible in part for potassium's protective mechanism against development of hypertension.

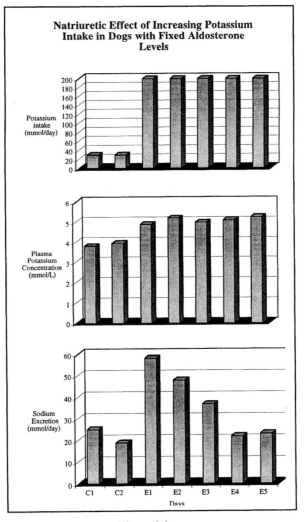

**Figure 9.2**

*Shown here are the responses of plasma potassium concentration and sodium excretion to an increase in potassium intake in adrenalectomized dogs maintained on fixed aldosterone replacement. From reference 162.*

# Renin Release

Renin is secreted from the juxtaglomerular (JG) cells, modified vascular smooth muscle cells lining the afferent arteriolar close to the glomerulus (for review see references 46, 163). Increased rates of renin release are associated with reductions in renal perfusion pressure (the baroreceptor mechanism), reductions in delivery of sodium and/or chloride to the macula densa region of the early distal nephron (the macula densa mechanism), and increases in the level of activity in sympathetic nervous system neurons innervating the juxtaglomerular cells (acting through beta adrenergic receptors). Renin release is inhibited by alpha adrenergic antagonists, angiotensin II, elevation of renal perfusion pressure, and by increases in rate of delivery of sodium and/or chloride to the macula densa region of the distal nephron. A growing body of evidence suggests that renin release is inversely related to intracellular calcium concentration in the juxtaglomerular cells. For example, Kurtz et al. directly demonstrated in juxtaglomerular cells that vasoconstrictors such as angiotensin II, nor-epinephrine and vasopressin increase intracellular calcium and inhibit renin secretion (164). In contrast, the calcium entry blocker verapamil decreases calcium concentration in the JG cells and elevates renin release. On the basis of these and similar findings by others, it has been proposed that calcium concentrations is the intracellular signal that regulates renin release through the baroreceptor mechanism, the macula densa mechanism, and the renal sympathetic nervous pathways (165). Under most conditions, the juxtaglomerular cells are receiving input from the macula densa mechanism, the baroreceptor mechanism, and the sympathetic nervous system simultaneously; the rate of renin release is finally determined by the intracellular calcium concentration that results from the integration of input signals by the juxtaglomerular cells.

Changes in potassium concentration in the plasma have the potential to affect renin release by several mechanisms. Elevation of potassium concentration within the physiological range (less than 8 mmol/L) causes relaxation of vascular smooth muscle and dilation of the renal vascular bed. These actions indicate that a reduction in intracellular calcium concentration in vascular smooth muscle results from such changes in potassium concentration, and consequently, the juxtaglomerular cells should respond with an increase in the rate of renin release. Elevation of potassium concentration within the physiological range also inhibits sodium reabsorption in portions of the nephron proximal to the macula densa, and elevate sodium delivery to the macula densa. Therefore, acting through the macula densa mechanism, raising potassium concentration in the plasma would be expected to lead to inhibition of renin release from the juxtaglomerular cells.

Under some experimental conditions stimulation of renin release by an acute elevation of potassium concentration can be observed. In experiments conducted in this laboratory potassium concentration was raised by intravenous infusion from 3.5 to 5.7 mmol/L in anesthetized dogs (155). Renal perfusion pressure was lowered in 10 mmHg steps from 120 to 60 mmHg. At each level of perfusion pressure renin release was measured. Elevation of potassium concentration had no significant effect on renin release until perfusion pressure was lowered below the autoregulatory range, below 80 mmHg. However, below the autoregulatory threshold, renin release in the high potassium group was approximately twice as great as in the control group. Significantly, the calcium entry blocker verapamil produced a very similar pattern of stimulation of renin release at perfusion pressures below the autoregulatory threshold. In this experimental setting, the direct effect of elevated potassium concentration on the juxtaglomerular cells resulted in a reduction in intracellular calcium concentration similar to that associated with the calcium entry blocker. At the same time, sodium excretion in the high potassium dogs was significantly elevated above that of the control groups. The natriuretic effect of hyperkalemia increased delivery of sodium to the macula densa, providing inhibitory input to the juxtaglomerular cells. The integrated outcome was dominated by the stimulatory influence contributed by the direct effect of potassium on the JG cells.

Over longer time courses, if the natriuresis induced by the increase in potassium intake is great enough to induce a significant negative sodium balance, the attendant volume depletion may contribute to stimulation of renin release. Bauer et al. found that in humans, plasma renin activity increased as potassium intake increased, probably secondary to the sodium or volume depletion induced by the high level of potassium intake (166).

Under different experimental conditions, potassium given both acutely and chronically can suppress renin secretion. In animal studies, it appears that the ability of potassium to suppress renin secretion is critically dependent on administration of the chloride along with potassium; if potassium is given as the bicarbonate salt, suppression of renin release may not be observed (167,168). Potassium appears to interact multiplicatively and negatively with sodium; in a study in rats Sealey et al. found that the suppression of plasma renin activity associated with elevating dietary potassium intake was much greater in animals on a low sodium diet than in animals than in rats on a normal intake of sodium (169). In man, Brunner et al. recorded approximately a 40% suppression of plasma renin activity following an increase in daily potassium (chloride) intake from 125 to 250 mmol/day (170). In cases such as these, the net inhibition may be explained by a predominant inhibitory effect of increased delivery of sodium to the macula densa overriding the stimulatory influence resulting from the increase in plasma potassium concentration acting on the JG cells directly.

Certainly, it is not always clear how the rate of renin release will be affected by a change in potassium intake. Therefore, the significance of an effect of potassium on renin release as a factor involved in the potential antihypertensive mechanism of potassium cannot be determined with certainty that this time.

# REDUCTION IN BLOOD PRESSURE BY ELEVATION OF POTASSIUM INTAKE IN EXPERIMENTAL HYPERTENSION

The effects of changes in dietary potassium intake on blood pressure regulation have been studied in many models of experimental hypertension. In the Dahl salt sensitive model of hypertension in the rat, the rate of rise of blood pressure associated with elevation of sodium intake was reduced in proportion to the molar ratio of sodium to potassium in the diet (171); Dahl reported that as potassium intake was elevated, the level of arterial pressure attained in the sodium-sensitive rats was reduced. Similar effects have been reported by others using the Dahl salt-sensitive rats and in other models of salt induced hypertension. Meneely and associates reported nearly 40 years ago that addition of a large amounts of potassium to a high sodium diet given to Sprague Dawley rats increased the survival of the animals (172,173); however, survival could not be correlated with a reduction in blood pressure associated with the increase in potassium intake. In the Wistar-Kyoto strain of spontaneously hypertensive rats, administration of a high potassium diet has been reported to partially protect against development of hypertension (174). Many studies conducted by Tobian et al. using the stroke prone spontaneously hypertensive rat model have shown significant reductions in severity of hypertension resulting from elevation of dietary potassium content from 0.7% to 2.1% (109). In the two kidney, one clip renal hypertensive form of hypertensive rat consuming a normal sodium intake, very high potassium intake resulting from addition of potassium chloride to the drinking water was associated with attenuation of the severity of hypertension (175).

These rat models are the standard tools used to study hypertension and its treatment. The fact that high levels of dietary potassium are effective in attenuating the rise in blood pressure in each model supports the clinical relevance of potassium's potential cardiovascular protective effect.

# REDUCTION IN BLOOD PRESSURE IN HYPERTENSIVE PATIENTS BY POTASSIUM SUPPLEMENTATION

The actions of potassium on the renal elements of the blood pressure control system, and the effects of dietary potassium on a broad range of models of experimental hypertension, provide the basis for study of potassium's clinical efficacy for treatment of hypertension. During the last 20 years several dozen clinical trials of been conducted utilizing a range of study designs. Not all of the results have been positive, but in general, potassium supplementation has been successful in producing at least a modest reduction in arterial pressure in hypertensive patients.

Recently, Whelton and He assessed the effects of supplementation with oral potassium on blood pressure using pooled analysis of published results of randomized, controlled trials (176). Because of the well known associations between blood pressure and other nutritional variables, some of which are highly correlated with potassium intake, only data from randomized, controlled trials of the effect of potassium in treating and preventing high blood pressure were included in the analysis. The English-language literature was searched for reports of such trials detailing the effects of potassium supplementation on blood pressure in humans, published before July, 1995. Inclusion in the analysis was confined to reports in which: 1) oral potassium intake was the only difference between the active treatment intervention (potassium supplementation) and the concurrent control group (using either parallel or crossover design), and, 2) information on reported mean blood pressure change following both active and control treatment was available. Thirty-three reports met these inclusion criteria. Mean baseline blood pressure and urinary electrolyte excretion were estimated by pooling average values for the potassium supplemented and control groups. The total number of study participants was 2,609. Twenty-one trials were conducted with hypertensive participants and 12 in normotensive subjects. Antihypertensive medications were concurrently administered in four of the 21 trials conducted in hypertensive patients. A crossover design was used in 21 trials and a parallel-arm design in 12. The dose of potassium prescribed for participants in the active treatment group was greater than 60 mmol/day in all but two trials, and greater than 100 mmol/day in 10; the median supplementation rate was 75 mmol/day.

An intervention-related trend toward a reduction in systolic blood pressure was observed in 26 of the 32 trials, and in 11 trials, the reduction in systolic pressure was statistically significant. Diastolic blood pressure trended towards a reduction in 24 of 33 trials, and in 11 of these, the reduction was statistically significant. Overall pooled estimates of effects of potassium on systolic and diastolic blood pressure were -4.4 and -2.4 mmHg, respectively (p < 0.001 for both values). When the analysis was restricted only to the 29 trials with a documented intervention-related net change in urinary potassium excretion of greater than 20 mmol/day, the potassium intervention effect on systolic pressure average -4.9 mmHg and the diastolic effect was -2.7 mmHg. The size estimates for reduction of systolic (-4.9 mmHg) and diastolic (-2.7 mmHg) levels were also higher when analyses were restricted to 29 trials in which no antihypertensive medications were administered.

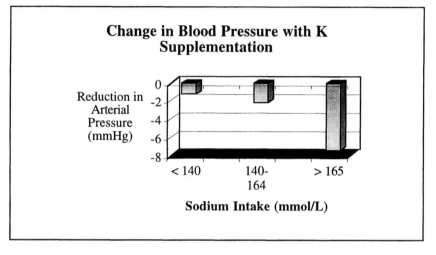

***Figure 9.3***

*The magnitude of change in mean arterial pressure was greater in studies reporting higher levels of sodium intake. From reference 177.*

Subgroup analyses revealed that a trend towards greater treatment-related reductions in systolic and diastolic blood pressure were expected at progressively higher levels of urinary sodium excretion during follow-up (p < 0.001). Linear regression analysis also identified a significant, independent positive relationship between 24-hour urinary sodium excretion and the corresponding net reductions associated with potassium supplementation in systolic and diastolic blood pressure. In participants whose urinary sodium excretion was less 140 mmol/day, the average reduction in mean arterial pressure following potassium supplementation was 1.2 mmHg; in subjects excreting sodium at a rate of 140-164 mmol/day, a 2.1 mmHg reduction in blood pressure was observed; and in the participants excreting more than 165 mmol/day a reduction of 7.3 mm Hg was associated with potassium supplementation (Figure 9.3).

At the higher levels of baseline sodium excretion, a dose-response relationship between 24 hour potassium excretion and the size of reduction in systolic and diastolic pressure was observed (p < 0.01). Also, a significant direct relationship between average pretreatment diastolic blood pressure and corresponding average treatment reduction of systolic pressure was noted. In addition, a significant difference between the responses of African-Americans and white participants was suggested; the average reduction in systolic blood pressure of the predominantly African-American groups was -5.6 mmHg, while in white groups it was -2.0 mmHg (p = 0.03) (Figure 9.4).

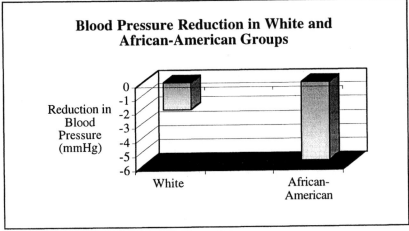

*Figure 9.4*

*Blood pressure reductions tend to be greater in predominantly African-American groups than in predominantly white groups. From reference 177.*

This statistically powerful study provides data supporting a causal relationship between potassium supplementation and reduction of blood pressure. Especially significant are: 1) the level of probability of the relationships between potassium administration and subsequent reduction in blood pressure of these randomized controlled clinical trials; 2) the narrow 95% confidence intervals around mean effect size estimates for the associations; 3) the degree to which the relationship has been replicated in varying settings and study designs; 4) presence of appropriate temporal sequences in prospective observational studies and clinical trials; 5) and the finding of a dose-response relationship between potassium and blood pressure reduction in observational and experimental studies. Even in the majority of the trials excluded from the meta-analysis conducted by these authors, the results are consistent with the hypothesis that potassium administration reduces blood pressure.

The average reduction in blood pressure in the 20 trials conducted in hypertensive subjects was of a sufficient magnitude (-4.4 and -2.5 mmHg for systolic and diastolic blood pressure, respectively) for the authors to support a recommendation that potassium supplementation be included in treatment of hypertensive patients, especially in African-American patients, and in those on a high level of sodium intake.

A recently completed study in normal subjects reinforced several of the main findings provided by Whelton et al. Morris and co-workers studied the effect of dietary potassium bicarbonate intake on salt-sensitivity in African-Americans and Caucasian (177). They analyze the blood pressure responses of 38 healthy normotensive men (24 African-American, 14 Caucasian) to changes in sodium intake in a study that lasted six weeks. The basal diets consumed for the entire six weeks study contained 15 mmol/day of sodium and 30 mmol/day of potassium. During the last four weeks, 250 mmol/day of sodium chloride was added; during the last three weeks, potassium was supplemented as potassium bicarbonate so that the total daily intake was either 70 or 120 mmol/day. Salt sensitivity was defined as an increase in mean arterial blood pressure of greater than or equal to 3 mmHg during salt loading; moderate sensitivity was considered as an increase in blood pressure between 3 and 10 mmHg, and severe sensitivity was defined as a blood pressure increase greater than or equal to 10 mmHg.

Salt loading combined with low potassium intake induced a significant increase in both systolic blood pressure and diastolic blood pressure in African-Americans as a group, but not in the Caucasian group. Salt sensitivity occurred in 79% of the African-Americans subjects and 36% of the whites (p < 0.02). Mean arterial pressure in the African-American group increased from 81.2 to 87.8 mmHg (p < 0.001), while in the white group the increase was from 79.9 to 81.9 mmHg (not significant). Supplemental potassium bicarbonate, 70 mmol/day, reduced the incidence of moderate salt sensitivity in African-Americans and whites; in the African-American group going from high salt with 30 mmol/day potassium to high salt, 70 mmol/day potassium, resulted in a decrease in mean arterial pressure from 89.2 to 85.3 mmHg (p < 0.01). In whites, the increase in potassium intake resulted in a change from 81.9 mmHg to 79.8 mmHg (not significant). In both groups, plasma potassium concentration increased 0.3 and 0.2 mmol/L, respectively; plasma renin activity also tended to increase in both groups with elevation of potassium intake. Body weight fell, by 0.4 and 0.6 kgs in the African-American and white groups, respectively.

Increasing potassium intake to 120 mmol/day abolished moderate sensitivity and reduce the occurrence of severe salt sensitivity in African-Americans. The impact of the elevation in potassium intake on frequency of occurrence of salt sensitivity and on the mean blood pressure change associated with elevation of salt intake are presented in Figure 9.5.

The authors also studied responses of subjects demonstrating moderate salt sensitivity to changes in potassium intake. In African-American group A, potassium intake was raised from 30 to 70 mmol/day for one week, then reduced to 30 mmol/day. During the one week of increased intake, mean arterial pressure fell by 3 mmHg, and then increased six mmHg when potassium intake was reduced to 30 mmol/day. Reduction in potassium intake was accompanied by a sustained decrease in urinary excretion of sodium. In African-American group B, potassium intake was increased from 30 to 70 mmol/day and maintained at that level for the duration of the experiment. Arterial blood pressure fell three to four mmHg and remained suppressed for the duration of the study. The subjects of African-American group C experienced an increase in potassium intake to 120 mmol/day, which was maintained for the duration of the study; the blood pressure of these subjects fell by approximately 5 mmHg and remained suppressed for the duration of the study.

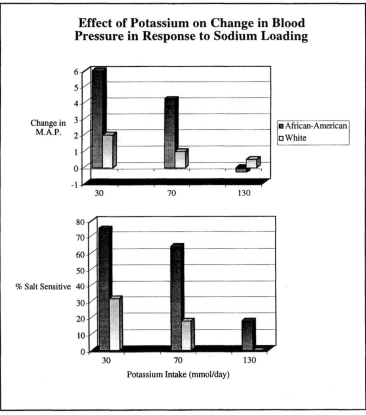

***Figure 9.5***

*Presented here are the effects of potassium intake on changes in mean arterial blood pressure (top) in response to increasing sodium intake from 15 to 250 mmol/day, and frequency of salt sensitivity (bottom) in African-Americans and whites. From reference 177.*

These observations suggest that in healthy normotensive African-Americans, but not in healthy normotensive Caucasians, when dietary potassium intake is at the low level consumed by many inhabitants of industrialized countries, 30 mmol/day, blood pressure is sensitive to the level of sodium in the diet. The findings further suggest that at this level of potassium intake, the majority of normotensive African-American men are salt sensitive, but only a minority of normotensive Caucasians are sensitive to salt. Increasing the dietary intake of potassium by only 40 mmol/day significantly attenuated the presser effect of salt in African-Americans. This reduced the incidence of moderate salt sensitivity in African-Americans and whites, and in each to a similar extent. Raising dietary potassium to a high-normal level of 120 mmol/day abolished moderate salt sensitivity and limited the occurrence of severe salt sensitivity. And only the moderately high level of potassium intake reduced the frequency of severe salt sensitivity in African-Americans to the same levels as those observed in whites consuming the diet containing 70 mmol/day. The studies in healthy normotensive men clearly demonstrate that dietary potassium modulates the blood pressure effect of dietary salt in both African-Americans and Caucasian, and determines whether salt sensitivity is present in most or only few of the African-Americans.

## BLOOD PRESSURE REDUCTION BY ELEVATION OF POTASSIUM INTAKE AND OTHER DIETARY MODIFICATIONS -- THE *DASH* TRIAL

The observation that vegetarians tend to have lower blood pressures than non-vegetarians has led to several trials of the effect vegetarian diets on blood pressure; replacing animal products with vegetable products generally has been shown to reduce blood pressure in both normotensive and hypertensive people. The vegetarian diet is believed to reduce blood pressure by a mechanism related to its high levels of fiber and minerals, and its reduced fat content. Most studies of the vegetarian effect have been observational in nature, and they have found frequently significant inverse associations of blood pressure with intakes of potassium, magnesium, calcium, fiber, and protein.

Recently, information from the investigations of vegetarians and blood pressure were incorporated in the design of a large multi-center trial entitled, Dietary Approaches To Stop Hypertension (DASH) (178). The trial was designed as a randomized feeding study to test the effects of dietary patterns on blood pressure, and as such, it was designed as a trial of dietary patterns rather than of individual nutrients. The study was conducted at several centers in the United States from 1994 to 1996.

Study subjects were 22 years of age or older who were not taking antihypertensive medication, with systolic blood pressure of less than 160 mmHg and the diastolic pressure of 80 to 95 mmHg. The cohort was made up of individuals from a wide range of socio-economic levels, with approximately two-thirds being members of minority populations. A total of 459 adults were enrolled in the study. For three weeks, the subjects were fed a control diet that was low in fruits, vegetables, and dairy products, with a fat content typical of the average diet in United States. The potassium, magnesium, and calcium levels of the control diet were close to the 25th percentile of U.S. dietary composition, and the macronutrient profile and fiber contents corresponded to average U.S. diets. After the three week run-in period, subjects were randomly assigned to receive for eight weeks either the control diet, a diet rich in fruits and vegetables, or a combination diet rich in fruits, vegetables, and low-fat dietary products that reduced saturated and total fat.

The fruit and vegetable diet provided potassium and magnesium at levels close to the 75th percentile of U.S. consumption, along with high amounts of fiber. This diet provided more fruits and vegetables and fewer snacks and sweets than the control diet, but was otherwise similar to it. The combination diet provided potassium, magnesium, and calcium at levels close to the 75th percentile of U.S. consumption, along with high amounts of fiber and protein. Sodium intake, approximately 3 g per day, and body weights were maintained a constant levels.

During the control period, the mean systolic and diastolic blood pressures were 131 and 85 mmHg, respectively. The combination diet reduced systolic and diastolic blood pressure by 5.5 and 3.0 mmHg more, respectively, than the control diet ($p < 0.001$ for each); the fruits and vegetable diet reduced systolic blood pressure by 2.8 mmHg ($p < 0.001$) and diastolic pressure by 1.1 mmHg more ($p = 0.07$) than the control diet (Figure 9.6).

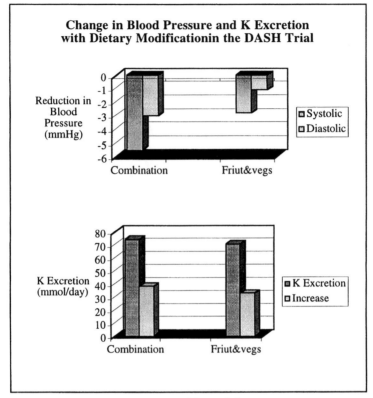

**Figure 9.6**

*Systolic and diastolic blood pressure (top) fell in both the fruits and vegetable group and the combination group. Potassium excretion (bottom) increased in both groups, by 39 mmol/day in the combination group and by 33 mmol/day in the fruits and vegetable group. From reference 178.*

Among the 133 subjects with hypertension (systolic pressure greater than 140 mmHg, diastolic pressure greater than 90 mmHg, or both), the combination diet reduced systolic and diastolic blood pressure by 11.4 and 5.5 mmHg more respectably than the control diet ($p < 0.001$ for each); among the 326 subjects without hypertension, the corresponding reductions were 3.5 mmHg ($p < 0.001$) and 2.1 mmHg ($p = 0.003$). Both in subjects with hypertension and in those without, the combination diet reduced blood pressure more than the fruit and vegetable or the control diet. In each pairwise contrast, subjects with hypertension had greater reductions in blood pressure than subjects without hypertension.

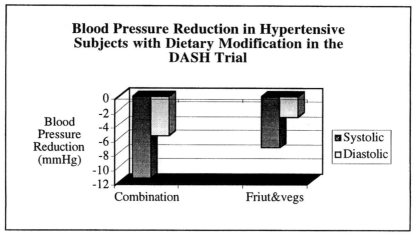

***Figure 9.7***

*Blood pressure reductions were greater in the hypertensive patients in the DASH trial. From reference 178.*

The blood pressure reductions with the combination and fruit and vegetable diets in hypertensive subjects are illustrated in Figure 9.7. The between-diet differences were greater in minority than in non-minority groups, although interaction between minority status and diet was not significant. There was no evidence of interaction between gender and diet.

Urinary potassium excretion increased substantially from the run-in phase to the intervention phase in the fruits-and-vegetables and combination groups; in the fruits and vegetable group it increased from 37 to 70 mmol/day, while in the combination diet group, potassium excretion rose from 36 to 75 mmol/day. Magnesium excretion increased only in the combination group. Urinary calcium excretion decreased in the control and the fruits-and-vegetable groups. In each group, urinary sodium excretion changed little between run-in and intervention phases.

Ambulatory blood pressure recordings were available for 345 of the subjects. The combination diet reduced mean 24-hour ambulatory systolic blood pressure by 4.5 mmHg more than the control diet, and diastolic pressure by 2.7 mmHg more (p < 0.001 for each). The corresponding reductions with the fruit-and-vegetables diet were 3.1 and 2.4 mmHg (p = 0.002).

The DASH trial demonstrated that blood pressure in adults can be affected favorably by adopting certain dietary patterns. A diet rich in fruits, vegetables, and low-fat dairy products and with reduced saturated and total fat lowered systolic blood and diastolic blood pressure. Of all of the constituents measured in the 24-hour urine samples, including potassium, magnesium, urea nitrogen, calcium, phosphorus, and sodium, only the increase in potassium excretion was consistently associated with reduction in blood pressure in the fruits-and-vegetables and combination diets. However, the trial was not designed to identify the effective and ineffective components of the diet, and therefore, a contribution of the potassium content of the diets to the reduction in blood pressure cannot be attributed with certainty.

The results of the DASH trial should be broadly applicable to the U.S. population. The cohort was demographically heterogeneous, with a range of entry blood pressures that included approximately 40% of U.S. adults. Approximately half of the subjects were women, 60 percent were African-American, and 37 percent had household incomes of less than $30,000 per year. Because the diets were made up of commonly available foods, the trial tested dietary patterns that the general U.S. population could easily adopt. The fruits and vegetable and combination diets included 8 to 10 servings per day of fruits and vegetables, approximately twice the average of 4.3 servings consumed by U.S. adults, and higher than the 5 to 7 servings per day recommended in the Dietary Guidelines for Americans. In the combination diet the 2.7 servings per day of dairy products are almost twice the current average consumption, 1.5 servings per day, but are within the dietary guideline recommendation of 2 to 3 servings per day.

The authors conclude that the DASH trial results have several clinical and public health implications:

*First, in view of the blood pressure reductions observed in the subjects without hypertension, the combination diet might be an effective nutritional approach to preventing hypertension. It is significant to note that the blood pressure reductions occurred without change in body weight, in sodium intake or alcohol consumption. Therefore, the combination diet may work synergistically with currently recommended measures for blood pressure control, including weight loss and reduction of sodium and alcohol intake.*

*Second, in the subjects with hypertension the reduction in blood pressure with the combination diet was similar in magnitude to that observed in trials of drug monotherapy for mild hypertension. Therefore, following the combination diet may be an effective alternative to step-one drug therapy for people with mild hypertension.*

*Third, adoption of the combination diet could potentially shift the population distribution of blood pressure downward, reducing the occurrence of blood pressure-related cardiovascular disease.*

# EVIDENCE FROM POPULATION STUDIES THAT HIGH DIETARY POTASSIUM INTAKE PROTECTS AGAINST DEVELOPMENT OF HYPERTENSION

During the last century, scores of studies have been conducted analyzing the blood pressures of groups living primitive, aboriginal lifestyles in Africa, Australia, South America, North America, and Asia. When eating the primitive diets the incidence of hypertension is no more than 1% in any of the groups, even though 5 to 10% live to their 60's or 70's. Once the group members begin using salt and eating processed foods they begin to develop hypertension and cardiovascular diseases at similar rates to the inhabitants of industrialized cultures, with 25 to 30% or more having elevated blood pressure (179,180). Therefore, these aboriginal groups do not appear to have a genetic resistance to development hypertension; their protection from the disease derives from their diet or lifestyle. Significantly, this list of hypertension-free groups includes some that have moderate rates of obesity (the Cuna Indians of Panama, reference 123), and some, such as the Yanomamo Indians of the Amazon rain forest (132), whose members experience lifelong intense emotional stress associated with nearly constant warfare that results in loss of property and women, humiliation, and the death of approximately one-third of the adult males in battle. The diets of all of these groups are made up primarily of vegetables and fruits, with less than one-third of the caloric intake coming from animal products. Consequently, the diets have much higher levels of potassium and fiber, and much lower levels of sodium and animal fats than the diets from industrialized cultures.

The differences in potassium and sodium content are striking; for example, Oliver and co-workers reported in a study of the Yanomamo Indians that the staple of their diet consisted of cooked banana, supplemented by regular additions of game, fish, insects, and wild vegetable foods (123). The tribe had had no regular access to sodium chloride when the study was conducted in 1975. Twenty-four hour excretion of sodium in adult males averaged 1 mmol, while potassium excretion averaged 152 mmol/day. Chloride excretion was less than 20 mmol/day. Plasma renin activity was elevated, averaging 13.1 ng/mL/hour (PRA), to a level expected in subjects on such a low intake of sodium; however, it is noteworthy that the high level of potassium intake did not suppress renin activity in the subjects. Urinary excretion of aldosterone was also found to be appropriately elevated, averaging 74.5 ug/24 hours. Blood pressure remained unchanged after the 10th year of age. The systolic and diastolic blood pressures during each decade of life for the male and female Indians are presented in Figure 9.8. Throughout adulthood systolic blood pressure in males average 101 to 108 mmHg, and diastolic pressure ranged from 63 to 69 mmHg.

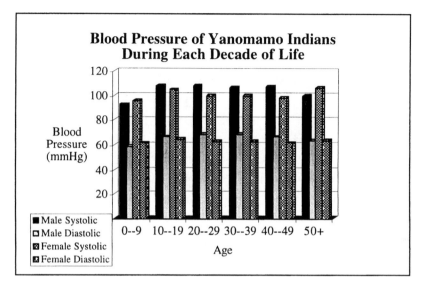

**Figure 9.8**

*Blood pressure of the Yanomamo Indians does not increase after the second decade of life. From reference 132.*

Analysis of regression of blood pressure on age revealed that the slope of the change in systolic pressure with age in males was -0.095, and in females it was -0.076; for males, the diastolic pressure slope was -0.010 and for females it was -0.032.

These observations of blood pressure in primitive groups are provocative, and they have given rise to speculation concerning the impact of dietary factors on population blood pressure. More recently, studies of large cohorts from several populations have been conducted utilizing standardized data collections and protocols, and intensive statistical analyses. In many cases the statistical power of these large studies enables going beyond speculation regarding relationships between dietary factors and blood pressure of populations. One of the first large studies was INTERSALT, an international collaborative study in which coordinated, standardized measurements of blood pressure and related factors were obtained from 10,000 participants age 20 to 59 years in 52 populations in 32 countries

(181). The groups included representatives from around the world, including the Yanomamo from Brazil, residents of Papua, New Guinea, Zimbabwe, from the countryside and cities of industrialized and developing nations. Included among the many findings was a highly significant inverse relationship between urinary potassium excretion and blood pressure; after correction for regression dilution bias and adjustment for age, gender, and other potential confounders, the pooled regression coefficient for the relationship between urinary potassium excretion and systolic and diastolic blood pressure in INTERSALT were -0.0446 and -0.0289 mmHg per mmol/day change in urinary potassium excretion, respectively. Based on this finding, a 50 mmol/day increase in potassium intake could be expected to reduce population blood pressure by 2.2 mmHg. Using the same population data, Rodriguez and co-workers analyzed the relationship between increase in population blood pressure with age and urinary excretion of sodium, potassium, body mass index and alcohol intake (182). Each of the INTERSALT populations was classified with regard to slope of the increase in systolic blood pressure with age; slope classification 0 was assigned to populations that showed 0 mmHg/year increase in blood pressure, category 1 corresponded to 0.17 mmHg/year, 2 = 0.33 mmHg/year, 3 = 0.50 mmHg/year, and 4 = 0.67 mmHg/year increase. The analyses of the populations' blood pressure slopes with age revealed a significant negative association between urinary potassium excretion and slope, and positive relations between blood pressure slope and urinary sodium excretion, sodium/potassium ratio, and reported alcohol consumption. Populations with zero slope had an average level of excretion of 75 mmol/day, populations with intermediate slopes (1 through 3) had urinary potassium levels from 54 to 57 mmol/day, and populations with the highest slope had the lowest average level of urinary potassium excretion, 49 mmol/day. For the sodium-potassium ratio, a graded positive relation with the slope of systolic blood pressure was also evident. Populations with 0 slope had a ratio 0.11; this ratio increased to 2.78 for slope category 1, 3.014 for slope 2, 3.13 for slope 3, and 4.20 for slope 4.

A similar study was conducted using a cohort from the United States in a study entitled National Health And Nutritional Examination Survey I

(NHANES I) (183).  McCarron et al. analyzed the relation of 17 nutrients to the blood pressure profile of adult participants (184).  Subjects were from 18 to 74 years of age, denying a history of hypertension and intentional modification to the diets.  10,372 individuals participated in the study that ran from 1971 to 1974.

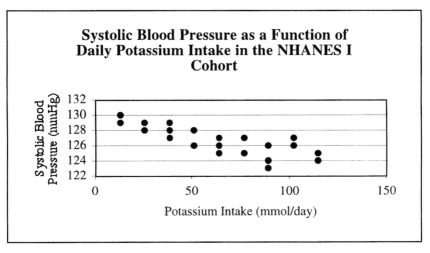

**Figure 9.9**

*The correlation between potassium intake and systolic blood pressure was highly significant in the NHANES I cohort.  From reference 184.*

When comparisons were made of nutrient intake and hypertension (defined as the upper 10% of blood pressures), with adjustments made for age, race, body mass index and gender, it was found that potassium, calcium, vitamin A and vitamin C were the nutrients whose intakes were significantly lower in hypertensive subjects (p < 0.001).  The potassium intake of the normotensive, lower 90% of the cohort averaged 57 mmol/day, and intake of the hypertensive, upper 10 percentile was 8.6% less, 52 mmol/day. Neither sodium intake, cholesterol consumption, nor phosphorous intake were consistently different among the various blood pressure and body mass index groups.  Increased consumption of potassium was negatively correlated (r = -0.461) with systolic blood pressure, as presented in Figure 9.9.

The authors applied several definitions of hypertension to the study population and, independent of effects of age, race, sex, body mass index, or alcohol consumption, lower levels of intake of for nutrients -- potassium, calcium, vitamin A, and vitamin C -- were statistically associated with hypertension. The authors conclude that there are predictable and crucial differences between individuals with high blood pressure and those with normal blood pressure, and that deficiencies rather than excesses are the principal nutritional patterns that characterized the hypertensive person in the United States. Furthermore, they concluded that reduced consumption of potassium and calcium are the primary nutritional markers of hypertension. And, in their analysis, diets low in sodium were found to be associated with higher blood pressure, while high sodium diets were associated with lowest blood pressures.

Data from the same study were analyzed by Frisancho and associates to determine the nature of blood pressure differences between African-Americans and whites, and its relationship to dietary sodium and potassium intake (185). A sample totaling 11,667 African-Americans and whites ranging from 20 to 74 years, who were not on any special diet or medication for hypertension were studied. The sample was divided into age, race, and gender groups.

In all age groups except among 25 to 34 year-old males and the 20 to 24 year-old females, the dietary intakes of sodium and potassium were found to be lower in African-Americans than in whites, even when the sodium and potassium intakes per 1,000 kcals were compared. Conversely, the sodium/potassium ratio among whites was lower than among African-Americans, indicating that the intake of potassium relative to sodium is less in African-Americans than in whites. Both systolic and diastolic blood pressures after the age of 35 years were significantly higher in African-Americans that in whites. These differences were not associated with concomitant differences in caloric intake, adiposity or body size.

On the basis of these results, it was concluded that African-Americans have a lower, not higher, intake of sodium than whites, a lower intake of potassium, and a significantly higher sodium/potassium ratio in their diet.

Although Frisancho did not attempt to associate the differences in dietary factors with hypertension, Watson and Langford, in a smaller study of 104 young African-American women in Jackson, Mississippi, reported a highly significant correlation between sodium/potassium ratio and systolic blood pressure ($p < 0.02$) (5,187). Potassium excretion was significantly and negatively associated with systolic blood pressure, while 24-hour sodium excretion showed no correlation to blood pressure.

The association of urinary sodium and potassium excretion with blood pressure was examined in the Rotterdam study, a population-based survey of men and women aged 55 and over (187). From the study population of 1,006, subjects were selected who had complete blood pressure and urinary data, who did not use antihypertensive drugs, and did not report themselves to be hypertensive. The mean age of the study population was 67.3 years, and mean blood pressure levels were 132.2 mmHg systolic and 70.5 mmHg diastolic. The mean 24-hour excretion rates were 119 mmol for sodium and 44 mmol for potassium. Dietary sodium/potassium ratio was 2.9.

Urinary potassium excretion, adjusted for age, gender, and body mass index, was inversely and independently associated with both systolic and diastolic blood pressure. The association with blood pressure was strong and was intensified after adjustment for sodium intake, -9.4 mmHg per 100 mmol/day for systolic and -4.9 mmHg per 100 mmol/day for diastolic blood pressure. For systolic blood pressure the association was more pronounced in men than in women (-11.3 vs -6.3 mmHg per 100 mmol). Urinary sodium excretion showed no independent relation with blood pressure, although after adjustment for potassium excretion, a 100 mmol/day increase in sodium was associated with a 2.2 mmHg increase in systolic pressure and a 0.8 mmHg increase in diastolic pressure; the association was significant only for the relationship between sodium excretion and systolic blood pressure in men. These observations suggest that blood pressure regulation may be especially sensitive to potassium intake in elderly subjects such as those in the Rotterdam cohort.

# SUMMARY

Experimental studies have demonstrated that elevation of potassium concentration in the blood affects elements of renal function in ways that are known to be associated with long-term reductions in blood pressure. In a wide range of animal models of hypertension, dietary potassium supplementation has been effective in reducing blood pressure and/or prolonging survival. Potassium supplementation, in many but not all studies, reduces blood pressure in hypertensive subjects, and dietary modifications that increased potassium intake were found to substantially reduce blood pressure in hypertensive and normotensive subjects. In several of the largest population studies of factors associated with hypertension, involving subjects from all parts of the world, potassium intake was reported to be inversely and strongly related to blood pressure. The magnitude of the effect is sufficiently great to warrant recommendation by the authors of some of the studies that potassium supplementation and dietary modification to a higher potassium intake be recommended for hypertensive patients, and for normotensive subjects to reduce their risk of developing hypertension.

# Chapter 10

# ARRHYTHMOGENIC SIGNIFICANCE OF HYPOKALEMIA

## POTASSIUM'S IMPACT ON ELECTROPHYSIOLOGICAL PROPERTIES OF MYOCARDIAL CELLS

## ELECTROCARDIOGRAPHIC ALTERATIONS WITH CHANGES IN POTASSIUM CONCENTRATION

## CLINICAL DATA RELATING HYPOKALEMIA TO ARRHYTHMIAS

## SUMMARY

## POTASSIUM'S IMPACT ON ELECTROPHYSIOLOGICAL PROPERTIES OF MYOCARDIAL CELLS

The ratio of potassium concentration in the cell to that in the extracellular fluid is a major determinant of the resting membrane potential of the cells of the myocardium (for review of myocardial cell electrophysiology see references 188-191). The relationship is expressed mathematically by the formula:

$$E_m = -61 \left[ \log \left\{ (r[K^+]_c + 0.01[Na^+]_c) / (r[K^+]_e + 0.01[Na^+]_e) \right\} \right]$$

Where *r* is the 3:2 active transport ratio of the sodium, potassium-ATPase, *0.01* is the relative membrane permeability of sodium to potassium, and the subscripts *c* and *e* refer to the cellular and extracellular concentrations, respectively. The normal concentrations of potassium and sodium in the extracellular fluid are 4.2 and 140 mmol/L, and the intracellular concentrations are 12 and 140 mmol/L, giving a calculated membrane potential of –85 mV (cell interior negative). Potassium diffusion out of the cell down its concentration gradient is largely responsible for the resting membrane potential, since sodium diffusion in the opposite direction is limited by the lower membrane permeability for sodium. The loss of potassium ions makes the interior of the cell more negative than the extracellular fluid, and a stable resting potential is reached when the interior of the cell becomes sufficiently negative to oppose the diffusion of positively charged potassium ions down the concentration gradient favoring its movement out of the cell.

In cardiac pacemaker cells the resting potential is short-lived. Once the cell has recovered from an action potential and has repolarized to the resting potential described by the equation presented above, sodium permeability of the membrane begins to increase, allowing sodium ions to diffuse into the cell, depolarizing the membrane. As the membrane potential becomes less negative, voltage sensitive sodium channels open more frequently allowing membrane potential to become even less negative. Voltage sensitive potassium channels also open and the outward potassium current opposes the depolarization arising from the influx of sodium ions. Once the threshold potential is reached, -60mV in cardiac cells, an increase in sodium permeability of several orders of magnitude within a few milliseconds leads to rapid depolarization of the membrane, the action potential. This increase in permeability is mediated by the opening of " fast channels", as the voltage-sensitive sodium channels were first described. The interior of the cell transiently becomes electropositive to the extracellular fluid, at which point membrane sodium permeability decreases drastically while potassium permeability rises. In cardiac cells the time required for repolarization is longer than in nerve or skeletal muscle cells because of the occurrence of a plateau of the membrane potential in the electropositive range. Following initial depolarization driven by the opening of the fast sodium channels, voltage sensitive calcium channels open, allowing entry of calcium ions and additional sodium ions from the extracellular space. These " slow channels " remain open for several hundred milliseconds during which the interior of the cell remains positive compared to the exterior, the intracellular calcium concentration is greatly elevated above resting levels, and the contractile mechanism is active. The plateau is terminated by the delayed opening of voltage-gated potassium channels that increase potassium conductance sufficiently to return membrane potential to the resting, hyperpolarized state.

The electrophysiological properties of the cardiac cell membrane are highly sensitive to changes in extracellular potassium concentration as presented in Table 10.1 (188).

*Table 10.1*
*Electrophysiological Properties of the Myocardial Cell Membrane Affected by Changes in Potassium Concentration*

|  | Hypokalemia | Hyperkalemia |
|---|---|---|
| *Resting membrane potential* | - | + |
| *Upstroke velocity (dV/dt) phase 0* | - | 0 or + |
| *Action potential duration* | - | + |
| *Refractory period* | - | + |
| *Threshold potential* | 0 | + |
| *Automaticity* | - | + |
| *Conductivity* | - 0 + | - |

*- decrease, + increase,. 0 no change.*

Hypokalemia will tend to hyperpolarize the resting potential according to the relationship described in the equation presented above. If this were the only effect on the electrophysiological properties of the membrane, automaticity and excitability would be reduced in hypokalemia; however, the initial hyperpolarization of the resting potential removes some of the normal suppression of activation of the sodium channels, thereby increasing membrane excitability. Consequently, in the presence of hypokalemia an increase in the rate of spontaneous diastolic depolarization or phase four of the action potential is observed. As a result, the membrane potential reaches the threshold value more quickly, and there is an increase in membrane automaticity. In addition, because the value of the resting potential is a determinant of the upstroke velocity or the rate of depolarization of phase zero of the action potential, hyperpolarization associated with hypokalemia increases the upstroke velocity of phase zero. This, in turn, increases the velocity of impulse conduction through the myocardium. Hyperkalemia is associate with changes in the opposite direction; reductions in impulse formation or automaticity of the pacemaker tissue is observed, as well as a slowing or block of impulse conduction throughout the myocardium.

Hypokalemia is also associated with the a prolongation of the depolarized plateau phase of the action potential and delayed ventricular repolarization. Recall that the plateau phase ends when potassium permeability increases allowing potassium ions to move out of the cell, driven by the favorable electrochemical gradient. The permeability of the membrane to potassium appears to be reduced by reductions in extracellular potassium concentration. Therefore, in hypokalemia potassium permeability is reduced and the rate of repolarization is slowed. The delay in repolarization is very important clinically in that it prolongs the duration of the action potential and the relative refractory state.

# ELECTROCARDIOGRAPHIC ALTERATIONS WITH CHANGES IN POTASSIUM CONCENTRATION

The electrocardiogram is a reflection of the electrical events in the myocardium. The P wave represents depolarization of the atrium, the QRS complex represents ventricular depolarization, and the ST segment and the T and U waves represent ventricular and Purkinje fiber repolarization, respectively. Hypokalemia produces characteristic changes in the ECG that can be related to the changes in the action potential (188). In the presence of hypokalemia, there is lengthening of the QT interval, flattening of the T wave, and development of a U wave indicating prolongation of repolarization. When plasma potassium concentration falls to less than 3.0 mmol/L, increased amplitude of the P wave is observed, along with prolongation of the TR interval and widening of the QRS complex. When hyperkalemia is present, the QT interval shortens and the T wave becomes tall and peaked. The QRS may widen, indicating a slowing of intraventricular conduction, and intraventricular block may develop. The P wave generally decreases in amplitude and may disappear (sinus node arrest).

# CLINICAL DATA RELATING HYPOKALEMIA TO ARRHYTHMIAS

A variety of cardiac arrhythmias can be induced by hypokalemia, including premature atrial or ventricular beats, sinus bradycardia, paroxysmal atrial or junctional tachycardia, atrioventricular block, and even ventricular tachycardia or fibrillation (189). The mechanism by which arrhythmias are related to hypokalemia is incompletely understood, although it is likely that the enhancement of automaticity and the delayed ventricular repolarization work synergistically to predispose the myocardium to reentrant forms of arrhythmias. The likelihood of arrhythmias during potassium depletion is enhanced in a number of common clinical settings, including coronary ischemia, left ventricular hypertrophy, and the use of digitalis. Digitalis-induced arrhythmias can be seen with normal concentrations of drug when hypokalemia is present. When other risk factors are present in a patient, even mild hypokalemia at rest can be considered to be potentially dangerous, since stress-induced release of epinephrine can transiently lower plasma potassium concentration by an additional 1.0 mmol/L.

## Diuretic Treatment of Hypertension

Diuretic-treated hypertensive patients make up the majority of hypokalemic patients seen by physcians. The occurrence of arrhythmias and the relationship between hypokalemia and arrhythmias in this group have been studied extensively last 25 years. In 1981 Hollifield and Slaton (193) reported the results of study in which 38 patients with hypertension were treated with progressively increasing doses of hydrochlorothiazide up to 200 mg per day. Total body potassium fell from 4,107 to 3,269 mmol, while plasma potassium concentration fell from 4.5 mmol/L to 2.4 mmol/L. Ventricular premature contractions (VPCs) were recorded at rest and during exercise. Associated with the diuretic-induced reduction in potassium was an increase in VPCs from 0.6 to 2.6 per minute during static exercise and from 0.8 to 5.7 per minute during dynamic exercise. The frequency of VPCs was directly correlated with the decrease in serum potassium concentration resulting from the diuretics. Later, Hollifield reported a similar study in 35 patients given smaller doses of hydrochlorothiazide, up to 50 mg per day for 40 weeks (194). Plasma potassium concentration fell from 4.4 to 3.8 mmol/L. Again, VPC frequency was analyzed during both static and dynamic exercise before and after potassium depletion. During the control condition, static and dynamic exercise did not increase the frequency of ectopic activity, but during hypokalemia 29 of 38 patients had marked increases in VPCs during static exercise (1.8 vs 4.2 per minute) and dynamic exercise (1.8 vs 6.2 per minute). Once again, the author reported a significant correlation between frequency of ventricular arrhythmias and the change in serum potassium concentration induced by diuretic therapy, and between frequency of arrhythmias and plasma potassium concentration.

The relationship between potassium concentration and frequency of VPCs was analyzed in the Multiple Risk Factor Intervention Trial that included 12,866 men without symptomatic heart disease who were randomized to receive either special intervention with intensive risk modification or usual care (195). Hypertensive patients in the special intervention group were treated with either hydrochlorothiazide or chlorthalidone diuretics. Subjects in the special intervention group who had displayed abnormalities on the resting ECG at baseline had higher death rates from coronary artery disease than those of the usual care group who did not receive diuretics. Among 1,403 hypertensive men taking diuretics serum potassium was inversely related to VPC frequency; in this study a decrease in serum potassium concentration of 1.0 mmol/L was associated with a 28% increase in the number of VPCs (p < 0.05).

A Medical Research Council study of diuretic therapy for hypertension included 287 patients who underwent ambulatory electrocardiographic monitoring (196). After eight weeks of diuretic therapy there was no difference in the prevalence of ventricular premature contractions when compared with the control; however, after 24 months of therapy a significant increase in frequency of VPCs was observed in patients receiving thiazide diuretics compared to those treated with placebo. The frequency of VPCs was significantly and inversely related to serum potassium concentration.

Numerous other studies have failed to find an association between VPCs and serum potassium concentration. In general, the negative studies have been shorter in duration than the studies that reported a association between potassium concentration and arrhythmias. For example, in a report by Lumme and Jounela, 24 hypertensive patients were monitored before and after four weeks of diuretic therapy (197). In patients treated with hydrochlorothiazide, serum potassium concentration fell from 4.0 to 3.5 mmol/L, and those treated with indacrinone recorded a decrease from 3.9 to 3.3 mmol/L. An increase in frequency of ventricular arrhythmias was seen in four patients, each of whom had had baseline VPCs. Likewise, Madias and co-workers reported the results of the study in 20 patients treated with thiazide diuretics for four weeks (198). Serum potassium concentration fell from 4.4 to 3.0 mmol/L, and no increase frequency of arrhythmias was observed.

## Ventricular Premature Contractions in Myocardial Infarction

The potential relationship between serum potassium concentration and ventricular arrhythmias has been evaluated in a number of studies. The results are difficult to interpret for several reasons: first, many patients presenting with acute myocardial infarction also have sustained high levels of sympathetic nervous system activity, which can transiently lower serum potassium concentration by a large and variable extent;  second, patients with the most severe cardiac damage may have an increased risk of a arrhythmias, and may present in a state of circulatory shock of cardiac origin with associated acidosis and elevation of serum potassium concentration. Consequently, serum potassium measurements obtained when the patient presents with acute MI may not reflect the patient's potassium status prior to the event. Furthermore, the association of elevated potassium concentration with cardiogenic shock in patients with large, arrhythmogenic infarctions may obscure inverse correlations between  potassium concentration and frequency of ventricular arrhythmias in patients with less severe cardiac damage.

In spite of these difficulties, several investigators have reported an association of hypokalemia with ventricular arrhythmias in patients admitted for acute myocardial infarction. In a study of 590 patients admitted to coronary intensive care, some with acute myocardial infarction and others with unstable angina, arrhythmias or congestive heart failure, Kafka and associate reported that hypokalemia related to diuretic use was not associated with frequency of VPCs (200). However, when the analysis was restricted to patients with acute myocardial infarction, serum potassium was significantly lower in patients who had ventricular arrhythmias than in those who had no VPCs.  Dyckner et al. evaluated 676 patients who presented with acute myocardial infarction who had a blood sample for potassium measurement obtained immediately on admission to the coronary care unit (201). Of this group, 32% were receiving diuretic therapy, and 22% of these were hypokalemic (potassium concentration less than 3.6 mmol/L). Only 2% of patients not receiving diuretic therapy were hypokalemic. Patients who were hypokalemic, irrespective of diuretic use, had a higher incidence of VPCs post-infarction than those who were normokalemic (p < 0.01).

Several studies have been reported that have failed to document an association between serum potassium concentration and arrhythmias in patients with acute myocardial infarction. In a multicenter study involving therapy with timidol, Nordrehaug and Von der Lippe analyzed records of 1,074 patients admitted with acute myocardial infarction (202). They found no association between initial serum potassium concentration and frequency of ventricular arrhythmias. VPCs were observed in 43% of the 122 hypokalemic patients and in 36% of the 952 patients who had normal serum potassium concentrations. Solomon and Cole (203) reported on records from 152 patients admitted to coronary care with an acute myocardial infarction; hypokalemia was present in 14% of the patients, 56% of whom had VPCs. In patients with normal potassium concentration, 35 % had VPCs (not significantly different). Boyd and associates (204) retrospectively analyzed records of 103 patients admitted to coronary care with a variety of diagnoses and found no relationship between hypokalemia and occurrence of ventricular arrhythmias. 68% of hypokalemic patients (potassium concentration less than 3.5 mmol/L) had VPCs, while 51% of those with potassium concentrations greater than 3.5 mmol/L had premature ventricular beats.

# Ventricular Tachycardia and Fibrillation in Acute Myocardial Infarction

A convincing relationship between hypokalemia and incidence of severe ventricular arrhythmias emerges from several large clinical studies involving patients with acute myocardial infarction. Nordrehaug et al. (199) analyzed the probability of ventricular tachycardia in a series of 60 patients after myocardial infarction (Figure 10.1).

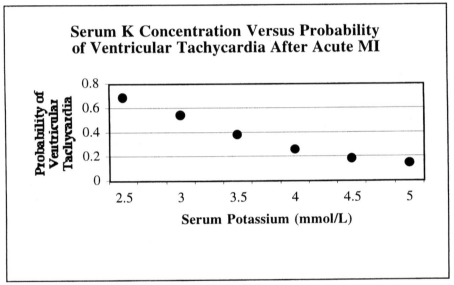

**Figure 10.1**

*In a study of 60 patients admitted with acute myocardial infarction, Nordrehaug reported a continuous inverse relationship between serum potassium concentration and risk of ventricular tachycardia. From reference 199.*

In 1,315 patients admitted to coronary intensive care, Hulting (205) reported in-hospital ventricular fibrillation occurred in 3.5% of patients, and that there was a close relationship between hypokalemia and the incidence of ventricular fibrillation. Ventricular fibrillation rates ranged from 8% in patients with potassium concentrations less than 3.5 mmol/L, to 1% in those with concentrations between 4.3 and 4.6 mmol/L. These data are presented in Figure 10.2. The author concluded that a serum potassium concentration less than 3.9 mmol/L increased risk of fibrillation fivefold ($p < 0.05$).

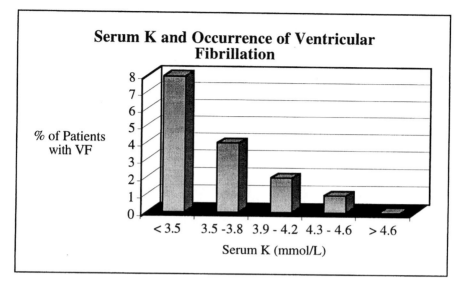

**Figure 10.2**

*Hulting observed that ventricular fibrillation was significantly and inversely related to serum potassium levels in coronary care patients. From reference 205.*

Solomon and Cole made similar observations in patients after myocardial infarction (203). In their sample, incidence of fibrillation was 25% if serum potassium concentration was less than 3.0 mmol/L, 15% when potassium was between 3.1 and 3.5 mmol/L, 9% between 3.6 and 4.0 mmol/L, and 5% when potassium concentration was between 4.1 and 4.5 mmol/L (Figure 10.3). Ventricular tachycardia or fibrillation occurred in 48% of patients with an initial serum potassium concentration less than 3.5 mmol/L, but in only 21% of patients with potassium concentrations greater than 3.5 mmol/L.

In a larger study of 117 to patients by the same group (206), ventricular tachycardia or fibrillation was reported in 29% of hypokalemic patients compared with 17% of patients with normal potassium concentration (p < 0.01). For ventricular fibrillation, 16% of those with hypokalemia experienced fibrillation, while 7% of those of normal potassium fibrillated (p < 0.01). 25% of patients with potassium concentrations < 3.0 mmol/L

experienced fibrillation, compared with 5% of those with concentrations
between 4.1 and 4.5 mmol/L.

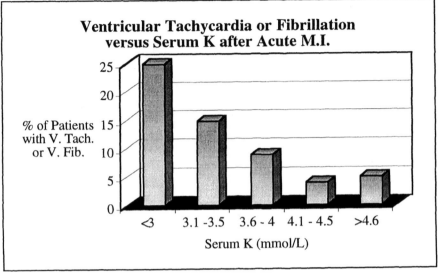

**Figure 10.3**

*Solomon and Cole presented evidence of a strongly significant inverse association between
serum potassium concentration and % of patients experiencing severe ventricular
arrhythmias after acute myocardial infarction. From reference 203.*

In the Norwegian timolol study by Nordrehaug and Von der Lippe
mentioned earlier (202), which involved 1,074 patients with acute
myocardial infarction admitted to the coronary care unit, ventricular
fibrillation occurred in 17.2% of hypokalemic patient, but in only 7.5% of
those with normal serum potassium concentration. In patients with
potassium concentration less than 3.0 mmol/L, ventricular fibrillation
occurred in 33%. In hypokalemic patients ventricular fibrillation occurred
earlier than in patients with normal potassium concentration;  in
hypokalemic patients who experienced ventricular fibrillation, 76%
fibrillated within two hours of admission. In patients with normal potassium
concentration who experienced fibrillation, 39% experienced it within the
first two hours.  In hypokalemic patients only 10% of ventricular
fibrillations occurred more than 12 hours after admission, whereas 42% of

the normokalemic patients fibrillated after more than 12 hours in the hospital.

In a study of 5,877 patients admitted for acute myocardial infarction, Johanssen and Dziamski (207) reported that incidence of ventricular fibrillation was increased 2.0 to 2.5 fold in hypokalemic patients. The relationship between hypokalemia and fibrillation persisted in both the presence and absence of prior to diuretic therapy ($p < 0.001$ for both).

## SUMMARY

Changes in extracellular potassium concentration can significantly impact electrophysiological properties of the myocardial cell membrane. Hypokalemia can hyperpolarize the resting potential, increase the rate of spontaneous depolarization during phase four, increase the rate of rise of the membrane potential during the upstroke of the action potential, prolong the plateau phase of depolarization, delay repolarization, and increase the duration of the refractory period. These changes increase automaticity of the myocardial cells and increase the rate of conduction of impulses through the myocardium. The mechanism by which arrhythmias are related to hypokalemia is incompletely understood, although it is likely that the enhancement of automaticity, increased conduction velocity and the delayed ventricular repolarization work synergistically to predispose the myocardium to reentrant forms of arrhythmias. Taken together, clinical studies support the existence of an strong, inverse relationship between plasma potassium concentration and frequency of ventricular tachycardia and fibrillation after myocardial infarction.

# Chapter 11

# MODERATE POTASSIUM DEPLETION IMPAIRS CARDIAC MECHANICAL FUNCTION

## CHRONIC HYPOKALEMIA AND LEFT VENTRICULAR FUNCTION IN DOGS

## CARDIAC FUNCTION RESPONSES TO MODERATE POTASSIUM DEPLETION IN NORMAL VOLUNTEERS

## SUMMARY

Changes in extracellular potassium concentration affect nearly all aspects of myocardial function. Reductions in potassium concentration alter the resting membrane potential, membrane conductance for sodium and potassium, repolarization time, relative refractory time, and conduction velocity. The arrhythmogenic consequences of these effects of potassium depletion have been discussed previously and are recognized to some extent by the medical community. However, the potential influence of hypokalemia on mechanical function of the heart has not been as thoroughly analyzed. Harrison and co-workers (207) observed severe cardiomyopathy in chronically potassium depleted rats that had plasma potassium concentrations of 2.2 mmol/L. The same group later reported suppressed peak velocity of contraction and isometric force generation in papillary muscles from severely hypokalemic (2.4 mmol/L) kittens (208). Galvez et al. (209) decreased potassium intake in dogs for six weeks, attaining a plasma concentration of approximately 2.0 mmol/L. Although they did not measure any direct indices of cardiac contractility, they did observe a 50% increase in basal cardiac output in the potassium depleted group. Brace and co-workers found that acute hypokalemia in dogs induced by hemodialysis resulted in increased left ventricular myocardial force, an effect they attributed to a ouabain-like effect of hypokalemia on sodium, potassium-ATPase of the myocytes (210).

It appears from these observations that although severe potassium depletion for periods of weeks results in cardiomyopathy and reduction in contractile force measured *in vitro*, more moderate, acutely induced potassium depletion may increase the strength of the heart. However, none of the studies provides information needed to determine if the degree of potassium depletion normally seen in patients has cardiac effect that are significant.

In this laboratory, we conducted two series of experiments designed to determine if moderate potassium depletion and hypokalemia have significant deleterious effects on mechanical function of the heart. The first series was conducted in dogs, and the second was performed using normal human volunteers.

## CHRONIC HYPOKALEMIA AND LEFT VENTRICULAR FUNCTION IN DOGS

Cardiac function was analyzed in a control group of 14 normokalemic dogs and a potassium depleted group of 13 similar dogs (211). The control group received a diet containing 50 mmol/day of sodium and potassium, while the hypokalemic group was given the same diet with altered electrolyte intake, 200 mmol/day of sodium and 10 mmol/day potassium. In addition, the hypokalemia group was given chlorthalidone orally for the first three days of the diet period. On the first day, 100 mg was given, on day two either 50 or 100 mg was given, depending on potassium excretion during the first day, and 50 mg was given on day three. On day four only diet was given.

Plasma potassium concentration in the deplete group was 3.2 mmol/L, which represents approximately an 8 to 10% reduction in total body potassium. Potassium concentration in the control group averaged 4.1 mmol/L. Cardiac function tests were conducted on day five.

The dogs were anesthetized, and the heart was instrumental for mechanical function measurement. Large bore catheters were inserted into the femoral artery and right atrial appendage and connected to a reservoir/pump containing 1.5 L of potassium-matched Tyrode's solution with 9% dextran.

Two types of function tests were performed. In Test I, a bolus injection of 2.5 ug/kg of epinephrine was rapidly injected i.v. Data were collected for a basal period and a 60 second response period after injection. In Test II, the response to a rapid, controlled increase in atrial pressure was analyzed (cardiac function curve). Blood was withdrawn into the pump through the femoral catheter and buffer solution was infused through the right atrial catheter until the hematocrit of the mixed blood and buffer solution in the pump were equal to that of the dog. Both the sympathetic and parasympathetic receptors were blocked prior to raising atrial pressure. A cardiac function curved consisted of a 30 second basal recording followed by rapid infusion (completed within 15 to 20 seconds) of the blood-buffer mixture until end-diastolic pressure was greater than 26 mmHg.

## Response to Epinephrine

Plasma potassium concentration of the two groups averaged 4.1 and 3.2 mmol/L. The inotrophic response to epinephrine, as assessed by maximal dP/dt and the peak rate of change of ejection power, was impaired by hypokalemia (Figure 11.1); in the normokalemic dogs the response of maximal dP/dt was 20% greater than the response in the hypokalemic dogs ($p < 0.03$). The maximal response of the peak rate of change of ejection power was 60% greater in the normokalemic group than the hypokalemic group ($p < 0.03$) (Figure 11.2).

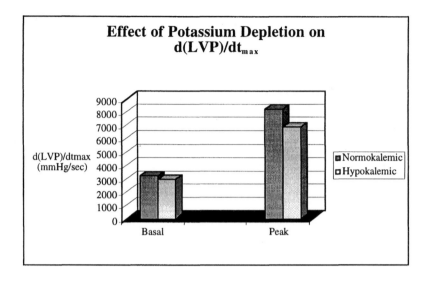

*Figure 11.1*

*Peak rate of change of left ventricular pressure (d(LVP)dt$_{max}$) during epinephrine stimulation was less in hypokalemia than during normokalemia. Basal function was unaffected. From reference. 211.*

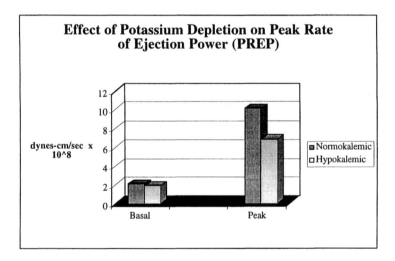

*Figure 11.2*

*Peak rate of ejection power was significantly less in the hypokalemic group than in the normokalemic group. From reference 211.*

The maximal response of peak systolic left ventricular pressure was 32% greater in the normokalemic than in the hypokalemic dogs (p < 0.003) (Figure 11.3), and the maximal response of isovolumetric relaxation, as assessed by the maximal rate of decline of left ventricular pressure, was 33% lower in the hypokalemic dogs (p < 0.02) . For each of these variables, basal values were not different in the two groups. Heart rate, cardiac index and stroke volume index increased from the basal levels in response to epinephrine in both groups;  however, there were no differences between groups with respect to either basal or peak values of these variables.  Nor were end-diastolic left ventricular pressure responses of the two groups different.

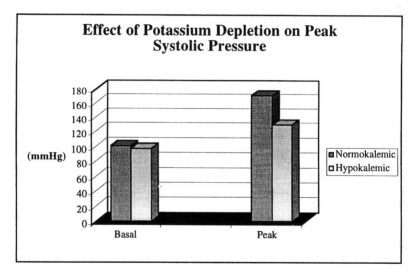

**Figure 11.3**

*Peak systolic pressure was significantly less in the hypokalemic group than in the normokalemic group.  From reference 211.*

## Cardiac Function Curves

Cardiac function curves were analyzed in subsets of eight normokalemic and eight hypokalemic dogs. Potassium concentrations of the two groups were 3.9 and 3.3 mmol/L, respectively.

End-diastolic volume index and end-systolic volume index increased in response to volume expansion in both groups, and there were no differences in these variables between the groups at any level of preload. Stroke volume index increased in response to volume expansion in both groups, although the response was significantly less in the hypokalemic group than in the control group. These data are presented in Figure 11.4.

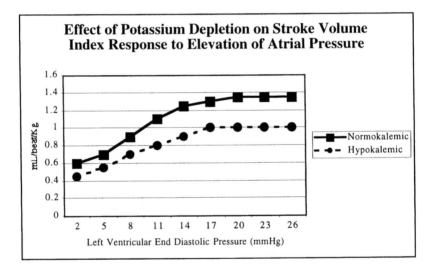

***Figure 11.4***
*Presented here are stroke volume index responses to rapid increases in preload of normokalemic and hypokalemic dogs. Potassium depletion and hypokalemia significantly reduced the index at high preload. From reference 212.*

In the control group stroke volume index increased from 0.60 to 1.40 mL/beat/kg in response to elevation of preload. The maximal stroke volume index of the hypokalemic group was 0.95 mL/beat/kg, 31% less than in the normokalemic group (p <   0.01).  Basal stroke volume index was not significantly different in the two groups, but as preload increased the stroke volume index response was attenuated by hypokalemia, so that there was a significant interaction effect of preload and potassium level.  The increase in cardiac index in response to preload was significantly lower in the hypokalemic group than in the control group.  In the control group cardiac index increased from 98 to 234 mL/min/kg during volume expansion, while in the hypokalemic group the maximal cardiac index was 26% less, 154 mL/min/kg (p < 0.01).  Basal cardiac index of the low potassium group (72 mL/min/kg) was not significantly different from that of the control dogs, but cardiac index responded less to increasing preload in the hypokalemic dogs.

In both groups, end-diastolic mean circumferential wall stress increased rapidly in response to preload, to a similar degree.  Since wall stress was not significantly affected by hypokalemia, the greater stroke volume index and cardiac index at high preload in the normal group cannot be attributed to either altered passive mechanical properties or differences in the experimental control of preload.

Peak systolic left ventricular pressure increased in both groups as preload increased.  The increases in pressure paralleled increases in cardiac index. Pressure was not significantly different between two groups at any individual preload, but at high preload peak systolic pressure tended to be lower in the hypokalemic group;  thus, the main effect of potassium was not significant, where as there was a significant interactive effect on pressure between preload and potassium.

The maximal filling rate index of the left ventricle increased rapidly in response to volume expansion in both groups, shown in Figure 11.5.  In the control group, filling rate rose from 15 to 42 mL/sec/kg at maximal preload, while in the hypokalemic group, filling rate increased to only a maximum of 23 mL/sec/kg, 51% lower than in normal group (p < 0.01).  Hypokalemia had a more severe impact at high preload than at basal levels (interaction effect, p < 0.01).  Left ventricular pressure at the time of maximal filling was not significantly different between the two groups, and thus was not responsible for the effect of hypokalemia on maximal filling.

This study was designed to determine whether or not chronic, moderate hypokalemia impairs mechanical function of the heart. The design reproduced the most common hypokalemic condition, that induced by diuretic therapy combined with high dietary sodium and low dietary potassium.

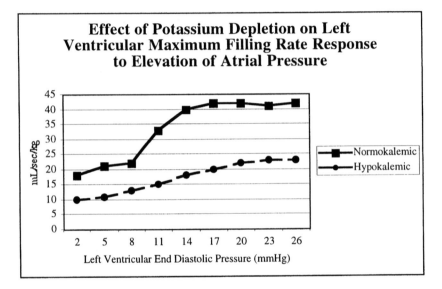

**Figure 11.5**

*Presented here are maximum left ventricular filling rate index responses to rapid increases in preload of normokalemic and hypokalemic dogs. Potassium depletion and hypokalemia significantly reduced the index at high preload. From reference 211.*

The design was effective in producing a plasma potassium concentration of 3.2 mmol/L in the experimental group, approximately 0.9 mmol/L less than the potassium concentration of the control group. We chose to study effects of hypokalemia on mechanical responses of the heart to two types of physiological stimuli; controlled increases in preload and elevation of circulating epinephrine concentration. The responses of the heart are closely related to modulation of cardiac performance by the main determinants of its physiological function -- variations in atrial pressure caused by changes in the rate of venous return, and increases in the level of sympathetic nervous system activity. These factors are influenced by behavioral stress, exercise and other physiological stressors. In addition, these mechanisms are employed to compensate for heart failure.

We found that hypokalemia strikingly limited the response of the myocardium to increases in preload and to epinephrine. Although the basal indices were not affected measurably, during chronic reduction in plasma potassium concentration, the maximal positive dP/dt and the peak rate of change of ejection power in response to epinephrine were reduced by 22% and 38%. Likewise, the effect of epinephrine on isovolumetric relaxation, assessed by the measurement of maximal negative dP/dt was reduced by 33% in hypokalemia. There were no significant differences in the end-diastolic left ventricular pressure between the groups; therefore, the lower responses of these indices to epinephrine were due to effects hypokalemia on cardiac contraction and relaxation rather than to effects of altered preload. The absence of effect of potassium on the cardiac index and stroke volume index responses to epinephrine is attributed to the lower sensitivity of these measures to the positive inotrophic influences catecholamines and their dependence on preload, which was identical in the two groups.

In response to controlled increases in preload, maximal stroke volume index was 31% less in the hypokalemic group than in the normokalemic group, and the maximal cardiac index response was decreased by 26% in the moderately potassium depleted group. Autonomic blockade was complete during preload increases, and therefore, the effects of hypokalemia on the cardiac responses to preload reflect direct effects on cardiac contractile performance rather than altered autonomic nervous system responses.

In the potassium depleted group, the maximal rate of filling of the left ventricle during increases in preload was reduced to 49% compared to the rate observed in the control group. This severe impairment of rapid filling was due primarily to decreases in active relaxation in the hypokalemic dogs; relaxation load during filling was the same in both groups at high preload, and there were no measurable differences in end-diastolic compliance (as assessed by either end-diastolic volume at controlled preload or end-diastolic wall stress), which, in any case, has little effect on rapid filling.

Our results differ markedly from numerous reports of increases in contractility during acute exposure *in vitro* to potassium-deficient solutions, and some reports of similar responses observed *in vivo*. Our data and those of other investigators demonstrate that chronic hypokalemia reduces contractility of the myocardium. As previously mentioned, Gunning and co-workers (208) observed major deficits in peak velocity of contraction and peak tension development in papillary muscles from severely potassium-deficient kittens. They also reported unchanged oxygen consumption despite reduced myocardial work, and interpreted this as a decrease in efficiency of oxidation metabolism. Although oxygen utilization was not measured in our experiment, such a phenomenon is consistent with our results in more clinically relevant hypokalemia; however, we observed no change in basal contractility, where as contractile function was impaired at all preloads in the severely potassium-deficient kittens. The report by Galvez et al. of increased cardiac output in long-term, severe potassium deficiency in dogs can be attributed to the extreme decrease in total peripheral resistance in their preparation, rather than to any change in contractility (209). Therefore, comparison of our results with reports involving severe hypokalemia *in vivo* indicates that as the severity of hypokalemia increases, its negative impact on cardiac function also increase.

Our observation of a dramatic effect of moderate hypokalemia on several aspects of cardiac mechanical function have several important clinical implications. First, hypokalemia and potassium depletion in the range of 3.0 to 3.4 mmol/L may not affect the unstressed function of the healthy heart, but may severely limit the ability of the myocardium to respond to an increase in preload or increased levels of sympathetic nervous system activity. Therefore, the ability of the heart to respond to stress and exercise may be reduced to a functionally significant degree by moderate hypokalemia in individuals with normal cardiac function. Second, the effect of hypokalemia on rapid filling would be expected to exacerbate the impairment that exists in the non-failing, hypertrophied heart. Third, patients with heart failure who have elevated preload and elevated levels of activity of the sympathetic nervous system would suffer further impairment of cardiac mechanical function due to moderate hypokalemia. This would be true at rest and in response to exercise or other stress. The deleterious effects of hypokalemia would be expected to be most severe in the patients with the most serious levels of heart disease.

# CARDIAC FUNCTION RESPONSES TO MODERATE POTASSIUM DEPLETION IN NORMAL VOLUNTEERS

The findings in the anesthetized, open chest canine experiments gave strong support to the possibility that moderate potassium depletion may significantly impair left ventricular mechanical function in clinical situations. We designed an additional experiment to test this possibility more directly in young adults (212). We recognized that in human subjects, we could not make all the measurements required to present a fully controlled study, as we had done in the dog experiments. The design was intended to be as close as possible to the one used previously in the animal studies, so that the results could be considered comparable to and possibly consistent with those of the preceding work. Accordingly, normal volunteers were studied during a potassium replete condition and during potassium depletion established by diuretics and a high sodium intake. In the animal studies we noted that the greatest effect of potassium depletion was observed when the heart was challenged, either by a rapid increase in preload or during epinephrine infusion. In the human studies, we chose to use the beta adrenergic agonist dobutamine given i.v. to challenge cardiac function. Left ventricular function was analyzed using Doppler and two dimensional echocardiographic techniques at rest and during intravenous dobutamine infusion.

Ten normal human volunteers were recruited for the study. They were given a thorough physical examination, and a resting 12-lead electrocardiogram was obtained. Subjects demonstrating any history, clinical, or ECG evidence of heart disease were not included in the study. All subjects gave informed written consent.

The study was designed to achieve a 1.0 mmol/L difference in plasma potassium concentration between the replete and deplete conditions in each subject. The subjects were divided into two groups of five. In Group I, the subjects were instructed to eat their normal diet and to take 12 potassium capsules per day, each capsule containing 8 mmol potassium chloride (96 mmol/day), for a period of seven days, after which cardiac function was analyzed. This was followed by another seven day period of potassium depletion. Approximately 1.25 mg/kg/day of chlorthalidone was given as 25 mg tablets, along with approximately 1.25 mmol/kg/day of sodium chloride given as the 1.0 g tablets. The sodium chloride was used to augment the kaliuresis and to prevent volume depletion. At the conclusion of the depletion period, cardiac function measurements were repeated. In Group II, the order of repletion-depletion was reversed.

Fasting baseline measurements of plasma potassium and sodium, blood pressure, and body weight were obtained in the morning between 8:00 a.m. and 10:00 a.m. before the start of the study, on several mornings thereafter, and on the seventh day of repletion or depletion. Blood for electrolytes measurements was drawn from the antecubital vein as the blood was freely flowing. During the potassium depletion period, measurements were made frequently so that the rate of depletion could be carefully monitored; if the rate of depletion was found to be too rapid, the doses of diuretic and sodium chloride were reduced.

Systolic and diastolic functions were evaluated by M-mode, two dimensional, and Doppler echocardiography. The maximal early (MVE) and late (MVA) left ventricular peak inflow velocities across the mitral valve were measured by Doppler techniques. Trans-mitral flow velocity was obtained from an apical window using the pulse wave Doppler technique by placing a 3 mm sample volume between the tips of the mitral valve leaflets. Settings for rejection and gain were recorded and held constant in the subjects for the potassium deplete and replete measurements. Isovolumetric relaxation time, deceleration time and the R-R interval for the cycle during which relaxation and deceleration were measured were obtained from the strip-chart record using standard techniques.

Two sets of measurements were made in the subject, one during the potassium repletion phase and the other during potassium depletion. During both phases, a resting or control set was recorded, followed by one or more sets made during dobutamine infusion. All recordings were obtained by a single experienced technician and every effort was made to keep the technique as consistent as possible.

Cardiac function was assessed beginning at 4:00 p.m. on the seventh day of the depletion -- repletion schedule. The subjects rested in a recumbent position for 10 minutes before the control cardiac function analyses were started. Six minutes were required to record the echocardiographic and Doppler data. When the control set was completed, an infusion pump was started, set to deliver dobutamine at a rate of 5 ug per kg per minute. The study design limited the infusion to rates less than those that resulted in ventricular arrhythmias, in systolic blood pressure elevation to more than 180 mmHg, and to increases in heart rate to more than 85% of the predicted maximum. Each rate of infusion was maintained for six minutes before cardiac function measurements were made. When one of the limits was approached, a second blood sample for electrolyte analysis was drawn after the measurement was completed, the infusion was stopped, the subject was monitored for 15 minutes, and then released. If the blood pressure, heart rate and ECG were within the study limits after the measurements, the next higher infusion rate was begun and continued for six minutes. One subject completed only the 5 ug/kg/min infusion rate, and nine completed the 10 ug/kg/min rate. In this subject group, systolic blood pressure approached the study limit in all subjects before the heart rate limit was attained. No ventricular arrhythmias were noted during the measurement.

Potassium concentration of the group was found to average 4.27 ± 0.12 mmol/L on the first visit to laboratory prior to taking supplements or diuretics. After potassium depletion, the group mean was 3.49 ± 0.12 mmol/L, while following repletion, the concentration rose to 4.57 ± 0.14 mmol/L. Blood pressure and heart rate data during cardiac function analyses are presented in Table 11.1.

*Table 11.1*
**Blood Pressure and Heart Rate during Potassium Repletion and Depletion**

| | Replete | | | Deplete | | |
|---|---|---|---|---|---|---|
| | **Systolic** mmHg | **Diastolic** mmHg | **Heart rate** beat/min | **Systolic** mmHg | **Diastolic** mmHg | **Heart rate** beat/min |
| **dobutamine** | | | | | | |
| **0 infusion** | 126±4 | 81±2 | 71±5 | 123±4 | 83±3 | 77±5 |
| **10 ug/kg** | 167±6 | 72±4 | 78±5 | 150±4 | 70±4 | 83±7 |
| **15 ug/kg** | 168±3 | 68±2 | 90±8 | 157±6 | 66±2 | 91±7 |

During the control measurements prior to dobutamine infusion, blood pressure averaged 126 ± 4 systolic and 81 ± 2 mmHg diastolic in the replete state, and 123 ± 4 systolic, 83 ± 3 mmHg diastolic in the deplete state. Following dobutamine infusion at 10 ug/kg/min, systolic blood pressure in the replete state was 167 ± 6 mmHg, significantly greater than the mean of 150 ± 4 mmHg in the deplete condition. Diastolic pressures were similar in the two conditions, 72 ± 4 and 70 ± 4 mmHg in the replete and deplete states, respectively. Heart rate was lower during repletion than depletion during the control measurements, 71 ± 5 beats/min versus 77 ± 4 beats/min, but the group means were not different during dobutamine infusion.

Atrial and ventricular dimensions during systole and diastole, at rest and during dobutamine infusion were strongly affected by dobutamine, but none was affected significantly by potassium status.

Doppler-derived measurements of mitral flow velocity, including MVE, MVA, isovolumetric relaxation time, deceleration time, and the R-R interval were obtained for each subject during repletion and depletion. MVE was significantly affected by potassium depletion ($p < 0.01$, Figure 11.6).

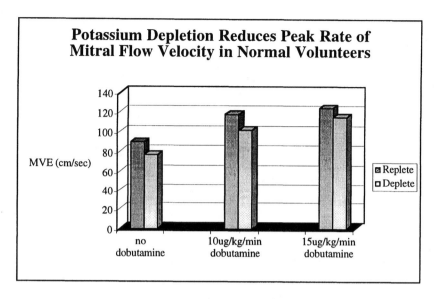

***Figure 11.6***
*In normal volunteers, MVE (peak rate of mitral flow), an indicator of active ventricular relaxation, was significantly reduced by moderate potassium depletion under basal conditions (no infusion of dobutamine), and during both levels of dobutamine infusion. From reference 212.*

With no dobutamine infusion, the group mean for MVE in the replete state was 89.5 ± 6.7 cm/sec, while in the deplete condition, the mean was 70.0 ± 4.9 cm/sec (p < 0.01). Infusion of dobutamine resulted in elevation of MVE in both conditions, although the mean value in the deplete condition remained significantly less than in the replete state; the value during infusion of 10 ug/kg/min dobutamine in the replete and deplete conditions were 117.8 ± 6.2 and 102.4 ± 7.0 cm/sec, respectively (p < 0.04). During infusion at the highest rate, 15 ug/kg/min, the replete and deplete means were 124. 3 ± 6.4 and 115.1 ± 4.6 cm/sec, respectively (p < 0.02).

The MVA and the ratio of MVE to MVA were not affected by potassium status. The isovolumetric relaxation time was significantly increased during depletion (p < 0.0001) (Figure 11.7). Deceleration time was also increased significantly by depletion.

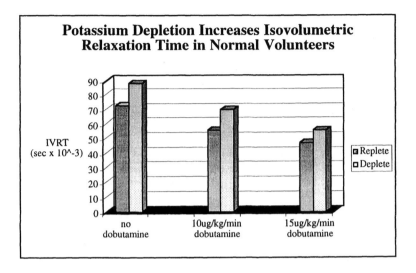

*Figure 11.7*

*In normal volunteers, IVRT (isovolumetric relaxation time), also an indicator of active ventricular relaxation, was significantly lengthened by moderate potassium depletion under basal conditions (no infusion of dobutamine), and during dobutamine infusion. From reference 212.*

In this study utilizing human volunteers, we did not observe significant differences between the potassium replete and deplete states in variables associated with contraction. However, MVE, which is the variable most closely corresponding to the peak filling rate index in the canine study, was strongly affected by potassium depletion. In the control condition prior to dobutamine infusion, MVE was 14% lower in subjects during depletion than during repletion. During infusion of dobutamine, the deplete values were 11% and 8% less than in the replete measurements. Isovolumetric relaxation time and deceleration time, which are also closely related to active relaxation of the myocardium, were significantly lengthened during potassium depletion. The finding of such a consistent effect of moderate potassium depletion on aspects of cardiac function associated with relaxation of the myocardium in healthy, young individuals, taken with the dramatic effect of a similar degree of potassium depletion observed in the canine study, strongly supports the hypothesis that potassium depletion may be a contributing factor to conditions characterized by impaired cardiac mechanical function in patients with potassium concentrations that are moderately reduced.

MVE is a function of the difference in pressure across the mitral valve immediately after opening. Therefore, it can be affected both by rapid reduction in left ventricular pressure resulting from active relaxation of the myocardium, and by the pressure in the left atrium. We recognized that a limitation of our study was that we could not measure directly left atrial pressure in our subjects, as we had in the animal study. Therefore, we cannot be certain that the decrease in MVE observed during potassium depletion was not do, in part, to a decrease in left atrial pressure. We did measure left atrial internal diameter to obtain an index related to left atrial pressure. And, we designed the study so that the potential for reduction in left atrial pressure due to diuretic administration would be minimized by the use of sodium chloride supplements along with chlorthalidone. Potassium depletion did not affect significantly atrial diameter; the differences between the group means were 1.7 mm or less during each of the measurements. Differences were not significant and were not correlated with changes observed MVE. Therefore, we propose that the changes in MVE observed in the human subjects were due primarily to changes in the active relaxation of the left ventricle.

Potassium depletion often coexists with magnesium deficiency, and severe, long-term magnesium deficiency is known to cause several forms of cardiac pathology, including arrhythmias and cardiomyopathy (213,214). Some diuretics, most notably those acting in the ascending limb of the loop of Henle, induce depletion of both elements. However, thiazide diuretics have a relatively weak effect on magnesium excretion. In acute studies in dogs (215) and rats (216), thiazides did not increase magnesium clearance, while results from human studies show a variable effect of thiazide diuretics (217-219). Therefore, we believe it is unlikely that in this study, the 7 day treatment with chlorthalidone induced magnesium wasting to an extent necessary to effect cardiac function.

# SUMMARY

It has been recognized for nearly a century that in various cardiac diseases, relaxation and diastolic function are impaired before contraction abnormalities become apparent (220-224). These early abnormalities in relaxation are commonly observed in several forms of hypertrophic and ischemic cardiomyopathy, and in other diseases including diabetic cardiomyopathy (225-231). In many such patients, hemodynamic abnormalities resulting in the clinical picture of heart failure are not due derangements of systolic function, particularly in the early stages of the disease. Instead, the functional defect may be due to active relaxation abnormalities. Many of the patient groups with demonstrated high risk levels for developing cardiac failure due to diastolic dysfunction are also at risk of developing moderate hypokalemia: the elderly, due to poor nutrition; the hypertensive, due to diuretic therapy; the African-American, due to dietary choices; and the diabetic. On the basis of the findings of this study and its predecessor in dogs, we propose that potassium depletion and hypokalemia may exacerbate heart failure associated with diastolic dysfunction in these groups. Furthermore, the results of the studies in animals and human subjects with normal cardiac function showing significant impairment of mechanical function due to moderate hypokalemia raise the possibility that those patients with left ventricular hypertrophy with or without signs of failure, and the elderly, are likely to be highly sensitive to the deleterious effects of hypokalemia.

The findings of the two studies presented here should be considered in evaluating the results of the recently completed RALES (Randomized Aldactone Evaluation Study) trial (60). The effect of spironolactone on severe heart failure was analyzed in a double-blind study involving 1,663 patients. Subjects were chosen who had no more than 35% left ventricular ejection fraction and were being treated with an angiotensin converting enzyme inhibitor, a loop diuretic, and in most cases, digoxin. The trial was discontinued early after a mean follow-up period of 24 months because interim analysis determined that spironolactone was efficacious; in the spironolactone group, relative risk of death compared to the control groups was 0.70 (p < 0.001). The reduction in risk of death among the patients in the spironolactone group was attributed to a reduced risk of death due to both worsening heart failure and sudden deaths from cardiac causes. In addition, the frequency of hospitalization for worsening heart failure was 35% lower in the spironolactone group than in the placebo group (relative risk, 0.65; p < 0.001), and the patients who received spironolactone had a significant improvement in the symptoms of heart failure, as assessed on the bases of the New York Heart Association functional classes (p < 0.001). The authors of the report attribute the beneficial effect of spironolactone to blocking the putative effects of aldosterone on formation of collagen. They do not report potassium concentrations of the subjects in either group, although they state that potassium concentration increased by 0.3 mmol/L in the spironolactone group over the course of treatment. We reported a prominent effect of less than a 1.0 mmol/L increase in potassium concentration to improve mechanical function of the left ventricle in normal dogs and healthy young volunteers. Blocking aldosterone's effect on potassium excretion by spironolactone administration would be expected to significantly increase plasma potassium concentration, which could have been responsible for the improvement in cardiac function in the heart failure patients. In addition to the direct benefit attributable to the effect of potassium on mechanical function of the ventricle, other well-established effects of potassium on sodium excretion and renin release could have contributed importantly to the improvement in clinical condition in patients treated with aldactone. The possibility that the increase in potassium concentration was responsible for the improvement of cardiac function in the RALES trial is tenable in light of our results, as well as those of others, and should be tested directly.

# Chapter 12

# CONCLUSION

## SUMMARY

## RECOMMENDATIONS

## CONCLUSIONS

The goal of this undertaking has been to present the most pertinent background information related to the question,

> *Can an elevation in potassium intake be protective against cardiovascular disease in individuals and in populations, and if so, should recommendation be made that potassium intake be increased in those at risk and in the general population?*

Information related to the question has accumulated for nearly a hundred years, from work in cellular physiology, from experimental studies in animals, from investigations in humans, and from population and epidemiological analyses. Because of the complexity of many of the topics, and the importance of integration of such a large, diverse body of information, the most important findings were presented here as a multichapter monograph rather than as a shorter review article. The central issues are summarized below, followed by recommendations based on their consideration.

# SUMMARY

The control system that maintains potassium balance is extremely effective in preventing changes in potassium concentration when intake of potassium is greater than normal. However, the system is much less effective in preventing reductions in potassium concentration when intake is reduced to less than the normal daily rate. Furthermore, the ineffectiveness in control as potassium intake falls below normal is exacerbated by high levels of sodium intake. These considerations are critical for understanding the relationship between potassium intake and the cardiovascular effects of the ion. Any relationship between a change in potassium intake and change in cardiovascular function would be expected to be more pronounced in the range of potassium intake below normal, particularly so if below-normal potassium intake were coupled with greater than normal sodium intake. Increasing potassium intake from normal to values greater than normal may not produce a measurable change in plasma potassium concentration or in the function of the cardiovascular system. However, if potassium intake were increased from well below normal to the normal rate, potassium concentration would be expected to rise measurably, and cardiovascular function would be more likely to be affected.

Changes in potassium concentration affect a number of central components of the blood pressure and sodium balance regulatory systems. These include the following effects of increases in extracellular potassium concentration:

> *Inhibition of sodium reabsorption in the ascending limb of the loop of Henle*
>
> *Dilation of the preglomerular vascular bed of the kidney, tending to elevated renal blood flow and GFR*
>
> *Inhibition of renin release*

Although the effects on these components have been studied primarily in short-term experiments, analyses of longer duration have demonstrated a sustained influence of changes in potassium on these systems. Therefore, this interaction between increases in potassium concentration with the central elements of the "pressure natriuresis - body fluid volume - blood pressure control system" may be responsible for the protective effect of high dietary potassium intake against the development of hypertension.

Results from laboratory experiments have demonstrated that changes in potassium concentration can affect the cells of the vascular system in ways that may provide an explanation for the vascular protective effects of diets containing a high potassium content. One of the earliest events contributing to formation of the atherosclerotic lesion is oxidation of LDL cholesterol in the subintima of the arteries by reactive oxygen species produced by monocytes, macrophages, and possibly endothelial cells and smooth muscle cells. In view of the inhibitory response to elevation of potassium concentration of free radical formation by monocytes and endothelial cells reported by McCabe et al., elevation of potassium concentration may be effective in inhibiting the path towards lesion development at this proximal point. Vascular smooth muscle cell migration and proliferation in the subintima are processes involved in maturation of the lesion, and the findings of Ma et al. of an inverse relationship between potassium concentration and migration and proliferation suggest that potassium's protective actions may include inhibition of the participation of smooth muscle cells in lesion formation as well. Potassium's ability to inhibit the thromboembolic consequences of advanced atherosclerotic lesions is supported by evidence from Lin et al.'s studies showing an inhibition by elevation of potassium concentration of thrombus formation in the coronary and carotid arteries of experimental animals models. Based on results of studies mentioned above and the work of others concerning the general mechanisms involved in vascular lesion formation, it is proposed that high levels of potassium in the diet inhibit the following mechanisms that could account for potassium's cardiovascular protective effects:

> *platelet aggregation and thrombus formation*
> *free radical formation and LDL oxidation*
> *vascular smooth muscle cell proliferation*
> *vascular smooth muscle cell migration*

These actions may provide protection against cardiovascular diseases that are related to lipid infiltration, foam cell formation and accumulation in the subintima, and thrombus and embolus formation.

Evidence from large population studies strongly implicates but does not prove an inverse association between dietary potassium intake and the risk of stroke. It is noteworthy that a strong protective effect of high potassium intake was observed in several studies in African-Americans, the segment of the U.S. population that has the highest risk of stroke. The association in man is supported by animal studies that clearly demonstrate that a high potassium intake provides protection from stroke in rat models. The relationship is further supported by the antithrombogenic effect of elevation of potassium concentration in the coronary and carotid arteries of experimental animals referred to in the preceding paragraph.

In a wide range of animal models of hypertension, dietary potassium supplementation has been effective in reducing blood pressure and/or prolonging survival. Potassium supplementation has been reported in many but not all studies to reduce blood pressure in hypertensive man, and dietary modification that increases potassium intake has been found to substantially reduce blood pressure in hypertensive and normotensive subjects. In several of the largest population studies of factors associated with hypertension, involving subjects from all parts of the world, potassium intake was reported to be inversely and strongly related to blood pressure. In many of the studies, the magnitude potassium's antihypertensive effect appeared to be comparable to that provided by step-one therapy with diuretics.

Changes in extracellular potassium concentration affect the electrophysiological properties of the myocardial cell membrane. Hypokalemia can alter these properties in ways that increase the automaticity of myocardial cells, increase the rate of conduction of impulses through the myocardium, and delay repolarization. These actions work synergistically to predispose the myocardium to reentrant forms of arrhythmias. Taken together, clinical studies support the existence of an inverse relationship between plasma potassium concentration and frequency of ventricular tachycardia and fibrillation after myocardial infarction.

Moderate potassium depletion induced by thiazide diuretics together with high sodium intake strongly impaired cardiac mechanical function in anesthetized dogs. The variables affected most significantly were those associated with the process of active relaxation that occurs during diastole. In healthy young adults, moderate potassium depletion of seven days duration induced by diuretics and high sodium intake also significantly impaired diastolic function, as estimated by peak rate of flow through the mitral the valve. The observed effect on diastolic function in these studies of normal man and animals may be of clinical importance in patients with heart failure.

# RECOMMENDATIONS

Consideration of these findings can lead to a number of recommendations concerning modifications in potassium intake for the general population, for persons at risk of developing cardiovascular disease, and recommendations for dietary intake and potassium supplementation for patients with cardiovascular diseases.

## Dietary Intake for Populations

Frequently, "normal" is considered to be equivalent to "ideal"; for potassium, the population average intake of 60 to 70 mmol/day is referred to as the normal value for healthy Americans. However, a high risk of hypertension, coronary artery disease and stroke are also considered to be "normal" for Americans as they enter middle age. Information from epidemiological and population studies, and from laboratory investigations, suggests that higher rates of daily intake may provide a reduction in risk of common cardiovascular diseases, and that cardiovascular risk may increase as potassium intake falls below 60 to 70 mmol/day. Therefore,

> *The minimum recommended daily intake for the*
> *general population should be no lower than 60*
> *mmol/day, the recommended intake should be greater*
> *than 100 mmol/day, and the ideal daily intake of*
> *potassium should be in the range consumed by*
> *primitive unacculturated populations, 250 mmol/day.*

To achieve an increase in intake of the population will require a concerted effort sustained for several decades. Success will require a commitment of resources by federal governments, international and national health-care organizations, private medical professional organizations, and medical universities. In addition, the food and beverage industries must be willing to participate in any effort to alter the potassium intake of the population.

The benefits of even a modest increase in population potassium intake are difficult to estimate. But based on the finding of studies reviewed in previous chapters, one can estimate that an increase in potassium intake of 20 to 30 mmol/day would significantly impact the population blood pressure and the risk of stroke, and possibly would reduce the incidence of coronary artery disease, potentially lethal cardiac arrhythmias, and congestive heart failure. The data appear to be available to calculate the expected cardiovascular health benefits associated with modest, feasible, increases in population potassium intake, and having such estimates will be essential for initiating a change in dietary recommendations.

## Minimum Recommended Value for Plasma Potassium Concentration

Plasma potassium concentration is considered to be "normal" if it lies between the 3.6 and 5.0 mmol/L. If a blood sample is collected properly and measured accurately, the potassium concentration in the blood of a healthy 70 kg adult consuming 60 to 70 mmol/day of potassium should not be below 4.0 mmol/L. If the subject was at rest and unstressed at the time the sample was drawn, and the measured concentration in the plasma is less than 4.0 mmol/L, it is likely the subject is consuming less than 60 mmol/day of potassium. Therefore,

> *The lower recommended limit of plasma potassium concentration should be 4.0 mmol/L, the concentration that is expected if the subject is consuming the minimum recommended daily intake. A confirmed reading less than 4.0 mmol/L should be considered as indicative of potassium depletion.*

## Potassium Intake for Athletes in Training

Especially for those who train and work in the heat, a high level of potassium intake is important for least two reasons. First, potassium can be lost at a rate of 10 mmol/hr or more in the sweat of subjects exercising or working vigorously in a hot environment. Loss at this rate for several hours on a daily basis can lead to significant potassium depletion in only a few weeks. Second, the cardiac performance that athletes depend on is probably limited to a significant degree by even mild potassium depletion. Therefore, it should be recommended that

> *Athletes should attain a high level of potassium intake, more than 60 mmol/day, during training by increasing their consumption of potassium-rich foods.*

## Potassium Intake for Patients at Risk of Developing Cardiovascular Disease

Patients at risk of developing hypertension, coronary artery disease, congestive heart failure, or stroke stand to benefit most from elevation of their potassium intake. Patients in these risk groups include those with family histories of the diseases, the overweight, the diabetic, the dyslipidemic, and the elderly.

> *Patients at risk of developing cardiovascular disease should consume at least 100 mmol/day of potassium, preferably from natural sources. They should receive counseling for the purpose of modifying their diets to contain as much potassium as possible.*

This type of dietary modification must be tailored to the needs of individuals, and to do so requires knowledge and understanding of dietetic issues. Therefore, physicians should encourage patients to seek counseling from a dietary professional.

## Potassium Intake for Patients with Cardiovascular Disease

Patients with hypertension, coronary artery disease, congestive heart failure, a history of cardiac arrhythmias, or of thromboembolic stroke may benefit from elevation of potassium intake.

> *For patients with cardiovascular disease, the physician should take steps to increase the patient's plasma potassium concentration to a value greater than the minimum recommended level of 4.0 mmol/L, and the daily intake of potassium to more than 100 mmol/day.*

Efforts should be made with those whose potassium concentration is less than the recommended level to adjust their medications, eliminating or reducing dosages whenever possible of potassium-wasting diuretics, replacing them when possible with potassium-sparing diuretics, or with angiotensin converting enzyme inhibitors. At the same time, the patient should be counseled to increase potassium intake from natural dietary sources; as mentioned above, this type of dietary modification may require input from a professional dietician.

If the patient's potassium concentration remains below 4.0 mmol/L, or if the patient is initially substantially potassium depleted as indicated by a plasma concentration less than 3.6 mmol/L, potassium supplements may be required to raise plasma concentration above the minimum recommended level. Taking potassium supplement entails some risk; before prescribing potassium supplements, the physician should carefully consider the patient's history and physical condition, with special consideration of renal function and concurrent use of potassium sparing diuretics, angiotensin converting enzyme inhibitors and angiotensin receptor antagonists, beta adrenergic blockers, and salt substitutes. The amount of supplementation given daily should be enough to increase the total daily intake of potassium to well over 100 mmol/day. Choice of the type of supplement should be made with consideration of the prospects for compliance. Therefore, the supplement that has the least side effects, provides the required daily amount of potassium in the fewest number of doses, and is the most affordable should be given preference. Potassium chloride or potassium bicarbonate appear to be equally effective as potassium supplements. Plasma potassium concentration should be monitored frequently, especially in the first weeks that the patient is on supplements, to guard against development of hyperkalemia.

# CONCLUSION

The information presented in the preceding chapters leaves little room for doubt about the importance of potassium in prevention of cardiovascular diseases. Elevation of plasma potassium concentration associated with the increased levels of dietary intake reduces the activity of cellular processes known to be critically important in formation of atherosclerotic lesions, reduces the sensitivity of platelet, alters elements of renal function in ways known to reduce blood pressure, inhibits thrombus formation at sites of arterial endothelial damage, inhibits formation of coronary arteriosclerosis in animal models, inhibits neointimal proliferation following angioplasty in coronary and carotid arteries of experimental animal models, lowers arterial blood pressure in animal models of hypertension, improves cardiac mechanical function in animals and in normal human volunteers, and inhibits thromboembolic stroke in experimental rat models. Furthermore, significant inverse relationships have been demonstrate between potassium intake or plasma concentration and population blood pressure, incidence of stroke, and incidence of potentially lethal cardiac arrhythmias. Finally, groups that have very high intake of dietary potassium have nearly complete protection against all of the major cardiovascular diseases that account for half of the deaths in industrialized cultures. This body of information provides emphatic support for the potential importance of high dietary potassium intake as a means for reducing risk of cardiovascular diseases. And, the information supports an affirmative answer to the initial question:

> *Yes, an elevation of plasma potassium concentration and intake can be protective against cardiovascular disease in individuals and in populations, and therefore, recommendations should be made that potassium intake be increased in those at risk and in the general population.*

The same information provides abundant evidence that potassium depletion and hypokalemia have significant, deleterious influences on many aspects of the cardiovascular system, influences that may cause or increase the risk of hypertension, atherosclerosis, heart failure, and thromboembolic conditions including stroke. Clustering of these serious cardiovascular diseases occurs in some groups that are known to be consumers of very low potassium diets, most notably, the African-Americans living in the southeastern United States. This clustering with potassium depletion may represent a syndrome that is important in understanding cardiovascular disease in African-Americans, and throughout the industrialized world.

Prevention of disease is always better than treatment, better in many respects. In the twentieth century we concentrated our attention and resources primarily on treatments for cardiovascular diseases, with a great deal of effectiveness. But in so doing, a mindset was created in the medical community that emphasized treatment almost to the exclusion of prevention.

As we begin the new century, we can clearly see that treatment will always remain too expensive monetarily and in terms of mortality to satisfactorily address the needs of the half of the population that will be afflicted by cardiovascular disease. And as I complete this work, I have no doubt that a large portion of that half of the population can prevent or delay development of cardiovascular afflictions by applying the findings of already completed scientific investigations to their own diets and life-styles. Support for the protective effects of diets with low saturated fat content is already strong. And now, the protective effect of high dietary potassium intake is also well supported scientifically. Other diet and lifestyle measures have been proposed as efficacious for prevention of cardiovascular disease, but additional information from well designed, controlled, impartial investigations will be required before they can be widely accepted. Until those data are in, the medical community will have to resist the temptation to recommend poorly supported approaches.

At this time we have the results and data required to strongly recommend dietary modification to increase potassium intake to more than 100 mmol/day for the general population and for patients at risk for development of cardiovascular disease. But making the recommendation will only be the first step; convincing the population to undertake the change in eating patterns will be challenging, and will require concerted actions by government, the medical community, and the food and beverage industries. The outcome promises to be well worth the investment.

# REFERENCES

1. Cerqueira MT, McMurry M, Fry W, Connor WE. The food and nutrient intakes of the Tarahumara Indians of Mexico. *Am J C Nutr.* 1979;32:905-915.
2. Hicks CS, Matters RF. The standard metabolism of the Australian aborigines. *Aust J Exp Biol Med Sci.* 1973;11:177-183.
3. Langford HG. Dietary potassium and hypertension: epidemiological data. *Ann Int Med.* 1983;948:770-772.
4. McCarron DA, Morris CD, Henry HJ, Stanton JL. Blood pressure and nutrient intake in the United States. *Science.* 1984;224:1392-1394.
5. Watson RL, Langford HG, Abernathy J, Barnes TY, Watson MJ. Urinary electrolytes, body weight and blood pressure, pooled cross-sectional results among four groups of adolescent females. *Hypertension Dallas.* 1980;2 (suppl 1):I-99-I-101.
6. Biagi B, Kubota T, Sohtell M, Giebisch G. Intracellular potentials in rabbit proximal tubules perfused *in vitro. Am J Physiol.* 1981;240(*Renal Fluid Electrolyte Physiol*):F200-F210.
7. Koeppen BM, Giebisch G. Mineralocorticoid regulation of sodium and potassium transport by the cortical collecting duct. In: Graves JS, ed. *Regulation and Development of Membrane Transport Processes. (Society of General Physiology Series).* Wiley, New York, 1984:89-104.
8. Koeppen BM, Biagi BA, Giebisch GH. Intracellular microelectrode characterization of the rabbit cortical collecting duct. *Am J Physiol.* 1983;244:F35-F47.
9. Proverbio F, Whittembury G. Cell electrical potential during enhanced Na extrusion in guinea-pig cortex slices. *J Physiol.* 1975;250:559-578.
10. Koeppen B, Giebisch G. Cellular electrophysiology of potassium transport in the mammalian cortical collecting tubule. *Pflügers Arch.* 1985;405: S143-S146.
11. Koeppen BM, Beyenbach KW, Helmann SI. Single-channel currents in renal tubules. *Am J Physiol.* 1984;247:F380-F384.
12. Palmer LG, Frindt G. Amiloride-sensitive Na channels from the apical membrane of the rat cortical collecting tubule. *Pro Natl. Acad Sci U.S.A.* 1987;3:2767-2770.
13. Sansom SC, O'Neil RG. Mineralocorticoid regulation of apical cell membrane $Na^+$ and $K^+$ transport of the cortical collecting duct. *Am J Physiol.* 1985;248:F858-F868.
14. Fujii Y, Katz A I. Direct $Na^+$, $K^+$ pump stimulation by $K^+$ in cortical collecting tubules: a mechanism for early renal K adaptation. *Am J Physiol.* 1989;257: F279-F284.

15. Bia MJ, DeFronzo RA. Extrarenal potassium homeostasis. *Am J Physiol.* 1981;240:F257-F268.

16. DeFronzo RA, Sherwin RS, Dillingham M, Hendler R, Tamborlane WV, Felig P. Influence of basal insulin and glucagon secretion on potassium and sodium metabolism. *J Clin Invest.* 1978;61:472-479.

17. Pan YJ, Young DB. Experimental aldosterone hypertension. *Hypertension.* 1982;4:279-287.

18. Young DB, Jackson TE. Effects of aldosterone on potassium distribution. *Am J Physiol.* 1982;243:R526-R530.

19. DeFronzo RA, Felig P, Ferrannini E, Wahren J. Effect of graded doses of insulin on splanchnic and peripheral potassium metabolism in man. *Am J Physiol.* 1980;238:E421-E427.

20. Bia MJ, Lu D, Tyler K, DeFronzo RA. β-adrenergic control of extrarenal potassium disposal---a $b_2$ mediated phenomenon. *Nephron.* 1986;43:117-122.

21. Young DB, Jackson TE, Tipayamontri U, Scott RE. Effect of sodium intake on steady-state potassium excretion. *Am J Physiol.* 1984;246:F772-F778.

22. Williams ME, Gervino EV, Rosa RM, Landsberg L, Young JB, Silva P, Epstein FH. Catecholamine modulation of potassium shifts during exercise. *N Engl J Med.* 1984;312:823-827.

23. Smith PL, McCabe RD. Potassium secretion by rabbit descending colon: effects of adrenergic stimuli. *Am J Physiol.* 1986;250:G432-G439.

24. Smith PL, Sullivan SK, McCabe RD. Potassium absorption and secretion by the intestinal epithelium. In: Lebenthal E, Duffey M eds. *Textbook of Secretory Diarrhea.* New York: Raven, 1990:109-118.

25. Blot-Chabaud M, Jaisser F, Bonvalet J P, Farman N. Effect of cell sodium on Na$^+$, K$^+$-ATPase-dependent sodium efflux in cortical collecting tubule of rabbits under different aldosterone status. *Biochim Biophys Acta.* 1990;1022:126-128.

26. Blot-Chabaud M, Wanstok F, Bonvalet JP, Farman N. Cell sodium-induced recruitment of Na$^+$, K$^+$-ATPase pumps in rabbit cortical collecting tubules is aldosterone-dependent. *J Biol Chem.* 1990;265:11676-11681.

27. El Mernissi G, Barlet-Bas C, Khadouri C, Cheval L, Marsy S, Doucet A. Short-term effect of aldosterone on vasopressin-sensitive adenylate cyclase in the rat collecting tubule. *Am J Physiol.* 1993;264:F821-F826.

28. Angeli M, Moura AM Worcel M. Interaction between aldosterone and vasopressin on vascular smooth muscle permeability to sodium. *J Steroid Biochem.* 1988;30:477-478.

29. Courty N, Farman N, Bonvalet JP, Blot-Chabaud M. Synergistic action of vasopressin and aldosterone on basolateral Na$^+$, K$^+$-ATPase in the cortical collecting duct. *J Membr Biol.* 1995;145:99-106.

30. Sterns RH. Oscillations of plasma K$^+$ and insulin during K$^+$ infusion in awake anephric dogs. *Am J Physiol.* 1982;243:F44-F52.

31. Furuya H, Tabei K, Muto S, Asano Y. Effect of insulin on potassium secretion in rabbit cortical collecting duct. *Am J Physiol.* 1992;262:F30-35.

32. Johnson JP, Jones DP, Wiesmann WP. Hormonal regulation of Na$^+$, K$^+$-ATPase in cultured epithelial cells. *Am J Physiol.* 1986;251:C186-C190.

33. Clauss W, Hoffmann B, Krattenmacher R, Van Driessche W. Current-noise analysis of Na absorption in the embryonic coprodeum: stimulation by aldosterone and thyroxine. *Am J Physiol.* 1993;265:R1100-R1108.

34. Geering K, Giradet M, Bron C, Kraehenbuhl JP, Rossier BC. Hormonal regulation of $Na^+$, $K^+$-ATPase biosynthesis in the toad bladder. Effect of aldosterone and 3, 5, 3'-triioco-L-thyronine. *J Biol Chem.* 1982;257: 10338-10343.

35. Pacha J, Pohlova I, Zemanova Z. Hypothyroidism affects the expression of electrogenic amiloride-sensitive sodium transport in rat colon. *Gastroenterology.* 1996;111:1551-1557.

36. Adrogue HJ, Madias NE. Changes in plasma potassium concentration during acute acid-base disturbances. *M J Med.* 71:456-464, 198.

37. Coplan NL, Gleim GW, Nicholas JA. Exercise related changes in serum catecholamines and potassium: effects of sustained exercise above and below lactate threshold. *Am Heart J.* 117:1070-1075, 1989.

38. Young DB, Srivastava N, Fitzovich DE, Kivlighn SD, Hamaguchi M. Potassium and catecholamine concentrations in the immediate post-exercise period. *Am J Med Sci.* 1992;304:150-153.

39. Young DB, Smith MJ, Jackson TE, Scott RE. Multiplicative interaction between angiotensin II and potassium concentration in stimulation of aldosterone. *Am J Physiol* 1984;247:E328-E335.

40. Young DB. The relationship between plasma potassium concentration and renal potassium excretion. *Am J Physiol.* 1982;242:F599-F603.

41. Young DB, Paulsen AW. Interrelated effects of aldosterone and plasma potassium concentration on potassium excretion. *Am J Physiol.* 1983;244:F28-F34.

42. Young DB. Analysis of long-term potassium regulation. *Endocrine Rev.* 1985;6:24-44.

43. Young DB. Quantitative analysis of aldosterone's role in potassium regulation. *Am J Physiol.* 1988;254:F810-F822.

44. Young DB, McCabe RD. Endocrine control of potassium balance. In: Fray JCS ed. *Handbook of Physiology: Section 7, The Endocrine System, vol III.* Oxford University Press, 2000:chapt 8, pp 306-330.

45. Squires RD, Huth EJ. Experimental potassium depletion in normal human subjects: relation of ionic intakes to renal conservation of potassium. *J Clin Invest.* 1959;38:1134-1140.

46. Laragh JH. Renin-angiotensin-aldosterone system for blood pressure and electrolyte homeostasis and it's involvement in hypertension, in congestive heart failure and in associated cardiovascular damage (myocardial infarction and stroke. *J Hum Hypertens.* 1995;9:385-90.

47. Young DB, McCaa RE, Pan YJ, Guyton AC. Effectiveness of aldosterone-sodium and potassium feedback control system. *Am J Physiol.* 1976;231:945-953.

48. Giebisch GH. Cell models of potassium transport in the renal tubule. In: Giebisch G ed., *Current Topics in Membrane and Transport.* Vol. 28. Orlando: Academic Press, 1987:133-183.

49. Wright FS, Giebisch G. Regulation of potassium excretion. In: DW Seldin and G Giebisch, eds. *The Kidney: Physiology and Pathophysiology.* Chap. 51, New York: Raven, 1985:1223-1249.

50. Fraley DS, Alder S. Correction of hyperkalemia by bicarbonate despite constant blood pH. *Kidney Int.* 1977;12:354-361.

51. Morgan TB, Davidson C. Hypokalemia and diuretics: an analysis of publications. *Br Med J.* 1980;280:905-912.

52. Siegel D, Hullet SB, Black D. Diuretics, serum and intracellular electrolyte levels, and arrhythmias in hypertensive men. *J Am Med Assoc.* 1992;267:1083-1089.

53. Schnaper HW, Freis ED, Friedman R. Potassium restoration in hypertensive patients made hypokalemic by hydrochlorothiazide *Arch Intern Med.* 1989;149:2677-2681.

54. Hropot M, Fowler N, Karlmark B, Giebisch G. Tubular actions of diuretics: distal effects on electrolyte transport and acidification. *Kidney Int.* 1985;28:477-489.

55. Young DB, McCaa RE. The role of the renin angiotensin system in potassium control. *Am J Physiol.* 1980;238:R359-363.

56. Frewin DB, Bartholomeusz RCA, Gaffney RD, Clampett AD, Chatterton BE. A comparison of the effects of lisinopril and hydrochlorothiazide on electrolyte balance in essential hypertension. *Br J Clin Pharmacol.* 1992;42:487-490.

57. Waeber B, Nussberger J, Brunner HR. Angiotensin converting enzyme inhibitors in hypertension. In: Laragh JH, Brenner BM eds. *Hypertension: Pathophysiology, Diagnosis and Management,* Second Edition. New York, Raven Press Ltd. 1995:2861-2876.

58. Dzau VJ, Colucci WS, Williams GH, Curfman G, Meggs L, Hollenberg NK. Sustained effectiveness of converting enzyme inhibition in patients with severe congestive heart failure. *N Engl J Med.* 1980;302:1373-1379.

59. Laragh JH. Spironolactone for treatment of hypertension or congestive heart failure: a review. *Excerpta Medica.* Princeton NJ, 1987.

60. Pitt B, Zannad F, Remme WJ, Cody R, Castaigue A, Perez A, Palensky J, Wittes J. The effect of spironolactone on morbidity and mortality in patients with severe heart failure. *New Engl J Med.* 1999;341:709-717.

61. Rose BD. Hypokalemia. In: *Clinical Physiology of Acid Base and Electrolyte Disorders,* Third Edition. New York: McGraw-Hill, 1989.

62. Epstein FH. Signs and symptoms of electrolyte disorders. In: Maxwell MH, Kleeman CR eds. *Clinical Disorders of Fluid and Electrolyte Metabolism,* 3rd edition. New York: McGraw-Hill, 1980.

63. Knochel JP. Neuromuscular manifestations of electrolyte disorders. *Am J Med.* 1982;72:521-535.

64. Dominic JA, Koch M, Guthrie GP, Galla JH. Primary aldosteronism presenting as myoglobinuric acute renal failure. *Arch Intern Med.* 1978;138:1433-1434.

65. Knochel JP, Schlein EM. On the mechanism of rhabdomyolysis in potassium depletion. *J Clin Invest.* 1972;51:1750-1758.

66. Knochel JP. Rhabdomyolysis and effects of potassium deficiency on muscle structure and function. *Cardiovasc Med.* 1978;3:247-251.

67. Hollander W Jr, Blythe WB. Nephropathy of potassium depletion. In: Strauss MD, Welt LB, eds. *Diseases of the Kidney,* Boston: Little, Brown, 1971.
68. Gordon P. Glucose intolerance with hypokalemia. *Diabetes.* 1972;22:544-546.
69. Helderman JH, Elahi D, Andersen DK. Prevention of glucose intolerance of thiazide diuretics by maintenance of body potassium. *Diabetes.* 1983;32:106-111.
70. Watten RH, Morgan FM, Songkhla Y. Water and electrolyte studies in cholera. *J Clin Invest.* 1959;38:1879-1886.
71. Collins KJ. The action of exogenous aldosterone on the secretion and composition of drug-induced sweat. *Clin Sci.* 1966;30:201-221.
72. Furman KI, Beer G. Dynamic changes in sweat electrolyte composition induced by heat stress as an indication of acclimatization and aldosterone activity. *Clin Sci.* 1963;24:7-12.
73. Carney S, Morgan T, Wilson M, Matthews G, Roberts R. Sodium restriction and thiazide diuretics in treatment of hypertension. *Med J Aust.* 1975;1:803-807.
74. Dyckner T, Wester PO. Extra- and intracellular potassium and magnesium, diuretics, and arrhythmias. In: Whang R, ed. *Potassium: Its Biologic Significance,* Boca Raton:CRC Press, 1983.
75. Dyckner T. Serum magnesium in acute myocardial infarction. Relation to arrhythmia. *Acta Med Scand.* 1980;201:59-66.
76. Textor SC, Bravo EL, Fouad FM, Tarazi RC. Hyperkalemia in azotemic patients during angiotensin converting enzyme inhibition and aldosterone reduction with captopril. *Am J Med.* 1982;73:719-725.
77. Sterns RH, Cox M, Feig PU, Singer I. Internal potassium balance and the control of plasma potassium concentration. *Medicine.* 1961;60:861-890.
78. Schribner BH, Burnell JM. Interpretation of the serum potassium concentration. *Metabolism.* 1956;5:468-480.
79. Nicolis GL, Kahn T, Sanchez A, Gabrilove JL. Glucose induced hyperkalemia in diabetic subjects. *Arch Intern Med.* 1981;141:49-53.
80. Steinberg D, Parthasarathy S, Carew TE, Khoo JC, Witztum JL. Beyond cholesterol. *N Engl J Med* 1989;320:915-924.
81. Steinberg D, Witztum JL. Lipoproteins and atherogenesis. *J Am Med Assoc.* 1990;264:3047-3052.
82. Ross R. Growth regulatory mechanisms and formation of the lesions of atherosclerosis. *Ann N Y Acad Sci.* 1995;748:1-6.
83. Hughes AD, Clunn GF, Refson J, Demolioy-Mason C. Platelet-derived growth factor (PDGF): action and mechanism in vascular smooth muscle. *Gen Pharmac.* 1996;27:1079-1089.
84. Krettek A, Fager G, Jernberg P, Ostergren-Lunden G, Lustig F. Quantitation of platelet-derived growth factor receptors in human arterial smooth muscle cells *in vitro*. *Arterioscler Thromb Vasc Biol.* 1997;17:2395-2404.
85. Nabel EG, Shum L, Pompili VJ, Yang ZY, San H, Shu HB, Liptay S. Direct transfer of transforming growth factor ß1 gene into arteries stimulates fibrocellular hyperplasia. *Proc Natl Acad Sci, USA.* 1993;90:10759-10763.

86. Ueno H, Li JJ, Masuda S, Qi Z, Yamamoto H, Takeshita A. Adenovirus-mediated expression of the secreted form of basic fibroblast growth factor (FGF-2) induces cellular proliferation and angiogenesis *in vivo*. *Arterioscler Thromb Vasc Biol.* 1997;17:2453-2460.

87. Dethlefsen SM, Shepro D, D'Amore PA. Arachidonic acid metabolites in bFGF-, PDGF-, and serum-stimulated vascular cell growth. *Exper Cell Res.* 1994;212:262-273.

88. Fafeur V, Jiang ZP, Bohlen P. Signal transduction by bFGF, but not TGF beta-1, involves arachidonic acid metabolism in endothelial cells. *J Cell Physiol.* 1991;149:277-283.

89. Sumiyoshi A, Asada Y, Marutsuka K, Hayashi T, Kisanuki A, Tsuneyoshi A, Sato Y. Platelets and intimal thickening. *Ann NY Acad Sci.* 1995;748:74-85.

90. Anderson PG. Restenosis: animal models and morphometric techniques in studies of the vascular response to injury. *Cardio Pathol.* 1992;1:263-278.

91. Jackson, CL. Animal models of restenosis. *Trends Cardiovasc Med.* 1994;4:122-130.

92. Schwartz RS, Holmes DR, Topol EJ. The restenosis paradigm revisited: an alliterative proposal for cellular mechanisms. *J Am Coll Cardiol.* 1992;20:1284-1293.

93. Lin H, Young DB. Interaction between plasma potassium and epinephrine on coronary thrombosis in dogs. *Circulation.* 1994;89:331-338.

94. McCabe RD, Backarich MA, Srivastava K, Young DB. Potassium inhibits free radical formation. *Hypertension Dallas.* 1994;24:77-82.

95. Ma G, Mamaril JLC, Young DB. Increased potassium concentration inhibits stimulation of vascular smooth muscle proliferation by PDGF-BB and bFGF. *Am J Hypertens.* 2000;13:1055-1060.

96. Canady KS, Ali-Osman F, Rubel EW. Extracellular potassium influences DNA and protein syntheses and glial fibrillary acidic protein expression in cultured glial cells. *Glia.* 1990;3:368-374.

97. Haddy FJ. Potassium effects on contraction in arterial smooth muscle mediated by Na$^+$, K$^+$-ATPase. *Fed Proc.* 1983;43:239-245.

98. Haddy FJ, Scott JB. Metabolically linked vasoactive chemicals in local regulation of blood flow. *Physiol Rev.* 1968;48:688-707.

99. Songu-Mize E, Caldwell RW, Baer PG. High and low dietary potassium effects on rat vascular sodium pump activity. *Proc Expr Biol Med USA.* 1987;186:280-287.

100. Sasaguri T, Masuda J, Shimokado K, Yokato T, Kosaka C, Fujishima M, Ogata J. Prostaglandins A and J arrest the cell cycle of cultured vascular smooth muscle cells without suppression of c-myc expression. *Exp Cell Res.* 1992;200:351-357.

101. McCabe RD, Young DB. Potassium inhibits cultured vascular smooth muscle proliferation. *Am J Hypertens.* 1994;7:346-350.

102. Jones AW. Content and fluxes of electrolytes. *In: Handbook of Physiology. The Cardiovascular System. Vascular Smooth Muscle.* Bethesda, MD. Am Physiol Soc. 1980: 253-300

103. Manuli MA, Edelman IS. Effect of high extracellular K$^+$ on Na$^+$-K$^+$-ATPase in cultured canine kidney cells. *Am J Physiol.* 1990;F227-F232.

104. Berridge MJ. Calcium signaling and cell proliferation. *Bioessays.* 1995;17:491-500.

105. Heitman J, Movva NR, Hall MN. Targets for cell cycle arrest by the immunosuppressant rapamycin in yeast. *Science.* 1991;253:905-909.

106. Ma G, Mason DP, Young DB. Inhibition of vascular smooth muscle cell migration by elevation of extracellular potassium concentration. *Hypertension.* 2000;35:948-951.

107. Stossel TP. From signal to pseudopod. *J Biol Chem.* 1989; 264:18261-18264.

108. Folts JD, Crowell EB, Rowe GG. Platelet aggregation in partially obstructed vessels and its elimination with aspirin. *Circulation.* 1976;54:365-370.

109. Tobian L. The protective effects of high potassium diets in hypertension, and the mechanisms by which high NaCl diets produce hypertension -- a personal view, *In:* Laragh H, Brenner BM eds. *Hypertension: Pathophysiology, Diagnosis, and Management,* Second Edition. New York: Raven Press, 1995.

110. Tobian L, Lange J, Ulm K, Wold L, Iwai J. Potassium reduces cerebral hemorrhage and death rate in hypertensive rats, even when blood pressure is not lowered. *Hypertension.* 1985;7 (suppl 2):I110-I114.

111. Todian L, Sugimoto T, Johnson MA, Hanlon S. High K diet protects against endothelial injury in stroke-prone SHR rats. *J Hypertens.* 1987;5(suppl 5) 263-265.

112. Khaw KT, Barrett-Conner E. Dietary potassium and stroke-associated mortality. *N Engl J Med.* 1987;316:235-240.

113. Lee CN, Reed DM, MacLean CJ, Yano K, Chiu D. Dietary potassium and stroke. *New Engl J Med.* 318:995, 1988.

114. Sasaki S, Zhang XH, Kesteloot H. Dietary sodium, potassium, saturated fat, alcohol, and stroke mortality. *Stroke.* 26:783-789, 1995.

115. Ascherio A, Rimm EB, Hernan MA, Giovannucci EL, Kawachi I, Stampfer MJ, Willet WC. Intake of potassium, magnesium, calcium, and fiber and risk of stroke among US men. *Circulation.* 1998;98:1198-1204.

116. Iso H, Stampler MJ, Manson JA, Rexrode K, Hennekens CH, Colditz GA, Speizer FE, Willet WC. Prospective study of calcium, potassium, and magnesium intake and risk of stroke in women. *Stroke.* 1999;30:1772-1779.

117. Franse LV, Pahor M, Bari MD, Somes GW, Cushman WC, Applegate WB. Hypokalemia associated with diuretic use and cardiovascular events in the systolic hypertension in the elderly program. *Hypertension.* 2000;35:1025-1030.

118. Fang J, Madhavan S, Alderman MH. Dietary potassium intake and stroke mortality. *Stroke.* 2000;31:1532-1537.

119. Ma G, Young DB, Clower BR. Inverse relationship between potassium intake and coronary artery disease in the cholesterol fed rabbit. *Am J Hypertens* 1999;12:821-825.

120. Page LB, Damon A, Moellerinng Jr RC. Antecedents of cardiovascular disease in six Solomon Islands societies. *Circulation.* 1974;49:1132-1146.

121. Truswell AS, Kennelly BM, Hansen JD, Lee RB. Blood pressures of Kung bushmen in northern Botswana. *Am Heart J.* 1972;84:5-12.

122. Lowenstein RW. Blood pressure in relation to age and sex in the tropics and subtropics. *Lancet.* 1961;1:389-392.

123. Kean BH. The blood pressure of the Cuna Indians. *Am J Tropical Med.* 1944;24:341-343.

124. Thomas WA. Health of a carnivorous race. A study of the Eskimo. *J Am Med Assoc.* 1927;88:1559-1560.

125. Donnison CP. Blood pressure in the African native. *Lancet.* 1929;1:6-7.

126. Murphy W. Some observations on blood pressures in humid tropics. *N Z Med J.* 1955;54:644-672.

127. Whyte HM. Body fat and blood pressure of natives in New Guinnea: reflections on essential hypertension. *Aust Ann Med.* 1958;7:36-46.

128. Kaminer B, Lutz WPW. Blood pressure in bushmen of the Kalahari desert. *Circulation.* 1960;289-295.

129. Connor WE, Cerqueira MT, Connor RW, Wallace RB, Malinow MR, Casdorph HR. The plasma lipids, lipoproteins, and the diet of the Tarahumara Indians of Mexico. *Am J Clin Nutr.* 1978; 31:1131-1142.

130. Williams AW. Blood pressure of Africans. *East Africa Med J.* 1941;18:109-117.

131. Morse WR, Beh YT. Blood pressure amongst aboriginal ethnic groups of Szechwam province, West China. *Lancet.* 1937;1:966-967.

132. Oliver WJ, Cohen EL, Neel JV. Blood pressure, sodium intake, and sodium related hormones in the Yanomamo Indians, a "no-salt" culture. *Circulation.* 1975;52:146-151.

133. Sacks FM, Rosner B, Kass EH. Blood pressure in vegetarians. *Am J Epidemiol.* 1974;100:390-398.

134. Groen JJ, Tijong KB, Koster M, Willebrands AF, Verdonck G, Pierloot M. The influence of nutrition and way of life on blood cholesterol and prevalence of hypertension and coronary heart disease among Trappist and Benedictine monks. *Am J Clin Nutr.* 1962;10:456-470.

135. Webster IW, Rawson GK. Health status of Seventh-Day Adventists. *Med J Aust.* 1979;1:417-420.

136. Ophir O, Peer G, Gilad J, Blum M, Aviram A. Low blood pressure in vegetarians. *Am J Clin Nutr.* 1988;48:806-810.

137. Gruntzig AR, Senning A, Siegenthaler WE. Nonoperative dilation of coronary artery stenosis: percutaneous transluminal coronary angioplasty. *N Engl J Med.* 1979;301:61-68.

138. Clowes AW, Reidy MA, Clowes MM: Mechanism of stenosis after arterial injury. *Lab Invest.* 1986;49:208-215.

139. Ma G, Young DB, Clower BR, Anderson PG, Lin H, Abide AM. High potassium intake inhibits neointima formation in the rat carotid artery balloon injury model. *Am J Hypertens.* 2000;13:1014-1020.

140. Ma G, Srivastava TN, Anderson PG, Grady AW, Skelton TN, Waterer HC Jr, Young DB. Inhibition of neointimal proliferation following balloon angioplasty in the swine coronary artery by high dietary potassium intake. *Am J Hypertens.* 2001; *in press.*

141. Karas SP, Gravasnis MB, Santonian EC, Robinson KA, Anderberg KA and King SB III. Coronary intimal proliferation after balloon injury and stenting in swine: an animal model of restenosis. *J Am Coll Cardiol.* 1992;10:467-474ed.

142. Willerson JT, Yao S-K, McNatt J, Benedict CR, Anderson HJ, Golino P, Murphree SS, Buja LM: Frequency and severity of cyclic flow alterations and platelet aggregation predict the severity of neointimal proliferation following experimental coronary stenosis and endothelial injury. *Proc Natl Acad Sci USA.* 1991;88:10624-10628.

143. Guyton AC, Hall JE, Coleman TG, Manning RD Jr and Norman RA Jr. The dominant role of the kidneys in long-term arterial pressure regulation in normal and hypertensive states. In: Laragh JH, Brenner BM eds. *Hypertension:Pathophysiology, Diagnosis, and Management.* New York: Raven, 1995: 1311-1326.

144. Coleman TG, Guyton AC, Young DB, DeClue JW, Norman RA Jr and Manning RD Jr. The role of the kidney in essential hypertension. *Clin Exp Pharm Physiol.* 1975;2:571-581.

145. Guyton AC, Cowley AW Jr, Young DB, Coleman TG, Hall JE, DeClue JW. Integration and control of circulatory function. In: Guyton AC, Cowley AW eds. *Cardiovascular Physiology II. International Review of Physiology.* Baltimore, MD: Univ. Park Press, 1976: 341-386.

146. Guyton AC. Circulatory Physiology III: Arterial Pressure and hypertension. WB Saunders, Philadelphia 1980.

147. Brandis M, Keyes J, Windhagger EE. Potassium induced inhibition of proximal tubular fluid reabsorption in rats. *Am J Physiol .* 1972;222:421-426.

148. Kirchner KA. Effects of acute potassium infusion on loop segment chloride reabsorption in the rat. *Am J Physiol.* 1983;244:F599-F605.

149. Stokes JB. Consequences of potassium recycling in the renal medulla. Effects on ion transport by the medullary thick ascending limb of Henle's loop. *J Clin Invest.* 1982;70:219-229.

150. Sufit CR, Jamison RL. Effect of acute potassium load on reabsorption of Henle's loop in the rat. *Am J Physiol.* 1983;245:F569-F576.

151. Scott JD, Emanuel D, Haddy F. Effect of potassium on renal vascular resistance and urine flow rate. *Am J Physiol.* 1975;228:305-308.

152. Beal AM, Buntz-Olsen QE, Clark RC, Cross RB, French TJ. Changes in renal hemodynamics and electrolyte excretion during acute hyperkalemia in conscious adrenalectomized sheep. *Quarterly J Exp Physiol.* 1975;60:207-221.

153. Shade RE, Davis JO, Johnson, JA, Witty RT. Effect of renal arterial infusion of sodium and potassium on renin secretion. *Circ Res.* 1972;31:719-727.

154. Vander AJ. Direct effects of potassium on renin secretion and renal function. *Am J Physiol.* 1970;219:455-459.

155. Lin H, Young DB, and Smith MJ Jr. Stimulation of renin release by hyperkalemia in the non-filtering kidney. *Am J Physiol.* 1991;260:F170-F176.

156. Lin H, Young DB. Impaired control of renal hemodynamics and renin release during hyperkalemia in rabbits. *Am J Physiol.* 1988;254:F704-F710.

157. Schneider GG, Lynch RE, Willis LR, Knox FG. The effect of potassium infusion on proximal sodium reabsorption and renin release in the dog. *Kidney Int.* 1972;2:197-202.

158. Webb CR, Bohr DF. A comparative and regional study of potassium induced relaxation in vascular smooth muscle. *J Comp Physiol.* 1980;135:357-363.

159. Anderson DK. Cell potential and the sodium-potassium pump in vascular smooth muscle. *Fed Proc.* 1976;35:1294-1297.

160. Baer PG, Navar LG, Guyton AC. Renal autoregulation, filtration rate and electrolyte excretion during vasodilation. *Am J Physiol.* 1970;219:619-625.

161. Addison WLT. The use of sodium chloride, potassium chloride, sodium bromide, and potassium bromide in cases of arterial hypertension which are amenable to potassium chloride. *Can Med Assoc J.* 1928;18:281-285.

162. Young DB, McCaa RE, Pan YJ, Guyton AC. The natriuretic and hypotensive effects of potassium. *Circ Res.* 1976; 38(suppl II):II-84-II-89.

163. Sealey JE, Laragh JH. The Renin-Angiotensin- Aldosterone System for Normal Regulation of Blood Pressure and Sodium and Potassium Homeostasis. In: Laragh JH, Brenner BM eds. *Hypertension:Pathophysiology, Diagnosis, and Management.* New York: Raven, 1995: 1797-1812.

164. Kurtz A, Pfeilschiffer J, Hutter A, Buhrle C, Nobling R, TaugnerR, Hackenthal E, Bauer C. Role of protein kinase C in inhibition of renin release caused by vasoconstrictors. *Am J Physiol.* 1986;250:C563-C571.

165. Fray JCS, Lush DJ, Park CB. Interrelationship of blood flow, juxtaglomerular cells, and hypertension: role of physical factors and calcium. *Am J Physiol.* 1986;251:R643-R662.

166. Bauer JH, Gauntner JW. Effect of potassium chloride on plasma renin activity and plasma aldosterone during sodium restriction in normal man. *Kidney Int.* 1979;15:286-293.

167. Kotchen TA, Galla JH, Like RG. Contribution of chloride to inhibition of plasma renin activity by NaCl in the rat. *Kidney Int.* 1978;13:201-207.

168. Kotchen TA, Krzyzaniak K, Ernst C, Galla JH, Luke RG. Inhibition of renin by HCl is related to chloride. *Am J Phsyiol.* 1980;239:F444-F450.

169. Sealy JE, Ckark I, Bull MB, Laragh JH. Potassium balance and the control of renin secretion. *J Clin Invest.* 1970;49:2119-2127.

170. Brunner HR, Baer L, Sealey JE, Ledingham JG, Laragh JH. The influence of potassium administration and potassium deprivation on plasma renin activity in normotensive and hypertensive subjects. *J Clin Invest.* 1970;49:2128-2138.

171. Dahl LK, Leitl G, Heine M. Influence of dietary potassium and sodium/potassium molar ratios on the development of salt hypertension. *J Exp Med.* 1971;136:318-330.

172. Meneely GR, Ball COT. 1958. Experimental epidemiology of chronic sodium chloride toxicity and the protective effect of potassium chloride. *Am J Med.* 1958;25:713-715.

173. Meneely GR, Ball COT, Youmans A. Chronic sodium toxicity: protective effect of potassium chloride. *Ann Int   Med.* 1957;47:263-271.

174. Sato Y, Ando K, Ogata E, Fuijta T. High potassium intake attenuates salt-induced acceleration of hypertension in SHR. *Am J Physiol.* 1991;260:21-26.

175. Suzuki H, Kondo K, Saruta T. Effect of potassium chloride on blood pressure in two-kidney one clip Goldblatt hypertensive rats. *Hypertension.* 1981;3:566-573.

176. Whelton PK, He J, Cutler JA, Brancati FL, Appel LJ, Follmann D, Klag MJ. Effects of oral potassium on blood pressure. *JAMA.* 1997;277:1624-1632.

177. Morris RC, Sebastian A, Forman A, Tanaka M, Schmidlin O. Normotensive salt sensitivity: effects of race and dietary potassium. *Hypertension.* 1999;33:18-23.

178. Appel LF, Moore TJ, Obarzanek E, Vollmer WM, Svetkey LP, Sacks FM, Bray GA, Vogt TM, Cutler JA, Windhauser MM, Lin PH, Karanja N. DASH collaraborative research group. A clinical trial of effects of dietary patterns on blood pressure. *N Engl J Med.* 1997;336:1117-1124.

179. Trowell H, Burkitt DP. Western Diseases: Their Emergence and Prevention. Edward Arnold, London. 1981

180. Page LB, Vandevert K, Nadetr N, Lubin N, Page JR. Blood pressure, diet and body form in traditional nomads of the Qash'qai tribe, southern Iran. *Acta Cardiol.* 1978;33:102-103.

181. The INTERSALT cooperative research group. Sodium, potassium, body mass, alcohol, and blood pressure: the INTERSALT study. *J Hypertens.* 1988;6(suppl 4):S584-S586.

182. Rodriguez BL, LaBarthe DR, Huang B, Lopez-Gomez J. Rise of blood pressure with age. New evidence of population differences. *Hypertension.* 1994;24:779-785.

183. Burt VL, Whelton P, Roccella EJ, Brown C, Cutler JA, Higgins M, Horan MJ, LaBarthe D. Prevalence of hypertension in the US population: results from the third National Health and Nutrition Examination Survey, 1988-1991. *Hypertension.* 1995;25:305-313.

184. McCarron DA, Morris CD, Henry HJ, Stanton JL. Blood pressure and nutrient intake in the United States. *Science, US.* 1984;224:1392-13948.

185. Frisancho AB, Leoinard WR, Bollettino LA. Blood pressure in blacks and whites and its relationship to dietary sodium and potassium intake. *J Chron Dis.* 1984;37:515-519.

186. Langford HG. Dietary potassium and hypertension: epidemiological data. *Ann Int Med.* 1983;948:770-772.

187. Geleinjnse JM, Witteman JCM, Hofman A, Grobbee DE. Electrolytes are associated with blood pressure at old age: the Rotterdam study. *J Hum Hypertens.* 1997;11:421-423.

188. Podrid PJ. Potassium and Ventricular Arrhythmias. *Am J Cardio.* 1990;65:33E-44E.

189. Brown H, Kozlowski R, Davey P. Physiology and Pharmacology of the Heart. Oxford Blackwell Scientific 1997.

190. DeMello WC, Janse MJ. Heart Cell Communication in Health and Disease. Boston. Kluwer Academic, 1998.

191. Jalife J. Basic Cardiac Electrophysiology for the Clinician. Armok NY. Futura Publishing, 1998.

192. Hollifield J, Slaton P. Thiazide Diuretics, hypokalemia and cardiac arrhythmias. *Acta Med Scand. [suppl]* 1991;647:67-73.

193. Hollifield JW. Potassium and magnesium abnormalities: diuretics and arrhythmias in hypertension. *Am J Med.* 1984:28-32.

194. Cohen JD, Neaton JD, Prineas RJ, Daniels KA and the Multiple Risk Factor Intervention Trial Research Group. Diuretics, serum potassium and ventricular ectopic activity. *JAMA.* 1982;60:548-554.

195. Medical Research Council. Working party on mild to moderate hypertension: ventricular extrasystole during thiazide treatment: Substudy of MRC mild hypertension trial. *Br Med J.* 1983;287:1249-1253.

196. Lumme JAJ, Jounela AJ. Cardiac arrhythmias in hypertensive outpatients on various diuretics. Correlation between incidence and serum potassium and magnesium levels. *Ann Clin Res.* 1986;18:186-190.

197. Madias JE, Madias NE, Bavras HP. Nonarrhythmogenicity of Diuretic Induced Hypokalemia. *Arch Intern Med.* 1984;144:2171-2176.

198. Nordrehaug JE, Johannessen KA, Von der Lippe G. Serum potassium concentration as a risk factor of ventricular arrhythmias early in acute myocardial infarction. *Circulation.* 1985;71:645-649.

199. Kafka H, Langevin L, Armstrong PW. Serum magnesium and potassium in acute myocardial infarction: influences on ventricular arrhythmia. *Arch Intern Med.* 1987;147:465-469.

200. Dyckner T, Helmers C, Wester PO. Cardiac dysrhythmias in patients with acute myocardial infarction. *Acta Med Scand.* 1987;216:127-132.

201. Nordrehaug JE, Von der Lippe G. Hypokalemia and ventricular fibrillation in acute myocardial infarction. *Br Heart J.* 1983;50:525-529.

202. Solomon RJ, Cole AG. Importance of potassium in patients with acute myocardial infarction. *Acta Med Scand. [suppl]* 1981;647:127-132.

203. Boyd JC, Bruns DE, DiMarco JP, Sugg K, Wills MR. Relationship of potassium and magnesium concentrations in serum to cardiac arrhythmias. *Clin Chem.* 1984;30:754-757.

204. Hulting J. In hospital ventricular fibrillation and its relation to serum potassium. *Acta Med Scand. [suppl]* 1981;647:109-116.

205. Nordrehaug JE. Malignant arrhythmias in relation to serum potassium values in patients with an acute myocardial infarction. *Acta Med Scand. [suppl]* 1981;647:101-107.

206. Johansson BW, Dziamski R. Malignant arrhythmias in acute myocardial infarction. Relationship to serum potassium and effect of selective and nonselective beta blockade. *Drugs.* 1984;28:suppl 1:77-85.

207. Harrison CE Jr, Novak LP, Connolly DC, Brown AL Jr. Adenosine-triphosphatase activity of cellular organelles in experimental potassium depletion

208. Gunning JF, Harrison CE Jr and Coleman HN III. The effects of chronic cardiomyopathy. J Lab Clin Med 75:185-196, 1970.

209. Galvez OG, Bay WH, Roberts BW, Ferris TF. The hemodynamic effects of potassium deficiency in the dog. *Circ Res.* 1977;40(suppl):I-11-I-16, 1977.

210. Brace RA, Anderson DK, Chen W-T, Scott JB, Haddy FJ. Local effects of hypokalemia on coronary resistance and myocardial contractile force. *Am J Physiol.* 1974;227:590-597.

211. Fitzovich DE, Hamaguchi H, Tull WB, Young DB. Chronic hypokalemia and the left ventricular responses to epinephrine and preload. *J Am Coll Cardiol.* 1991;18:1105-1111.

212. Srivastava N, Young DB. Moderate potassium depletion impairs diastolic function. *J Cardiac Failure.* 1995;1:195-200.

213. Bloom S. Magnesium deficiency cardiomyopathy. *Am J Cardiovasc Pathol.* 1988;2:7-17.

214. Massry SG. Role of hormonal and non-hormonal factors in the control of renal handling of magnesium. *Magnesium Bull.* 1981;3:277.

215. Eknoyan G, Suki WN, Martinez-Maldonado M. Effect of diuretics on urinary excretion of phosphate, calcium and magnesium in parathyroidectomized dogs. *J Lab Clin Med.* 1970;76:257.

216. Devane J, Ryan MP. Diuretics and magnesium excretion. *Magnesium Bull.* 1981;3:122-3.

217. McCollister RJ, Prasad AS, Doe RP, Flink EB. Normal renal magnesium clearance and the effect of water loading, chlorothiazide and ethanol on magnesium excretion: reactions of thiazide diuretics with parathyroid hormone and Vit. D: studies in patients with hypoparathyroidism. *J Clin Pharmacol.* 1972;51:1879-88.

218. Sullivan JM, Dluhy RG, Whacker WEC, Soloman HS, Williams GH, Somata JK. Interrelationships among thiazide diuretics and calcium, magnesium, sodium and potassium balance in normal and hypertensive man. *J Clin Pharmacol.* 1978;5:530-543.

219. Whacker WEC. The effect of hydrochlorothiazide on magnesium excretion. *J Clin Invest.* 1961;40:1086-7.

220. Katz LN. The role of the ventricular relaxation process in filling the ventricle. *Am J Physiol.* 1930;95:542-53.

221. Meijler FL, Brutsaert DL. Relaxation and diastole: introduction. *Eur J Cardiol.* 1978;7(suppl 1):1.

222. Dougherty AH, Naccarelli GV, Gray EL. Congestive heart failure with normal systolic function. *Am J Cardiol.* 1984;54:778-82.

223. Grossman W, McLaurin LP. Diastolic properties of the left ventricle. *Ann Int Med.* 1976;84:316-26.

224. Stauffer JC, Gaasch WH. Recognition and treatment of left ventricular diastolic dysfunction. *Prog Cardiovasc Dis.* 1990;32:319-32.

225. Ohsato K, Shimizu M, Shugihara N, Konishi K, Takeda R. Histopathological factors related to diastolic function in myocardial hypertrophy. *Jpn Circ J.* 1992;56:325-33.

226. Hanrath P, Mathey DG, Siegert R, Bleifeld W. Left ventricular relaxation and filling in different forms of left ventricular hypertrophy: an echocardiographic study. *Am J Cardiol.* 1980;45:15-23.

227. Sanderson JE, Traill TA, St John-Sutton MG, Brown DJ, Gibson DG, Goodwin JF. Left ventricular relaxation and filing in hypertrophy cardiomyopathy: an echocardiographic study. *Br Heart J.* 1978;40:496-501.

228. Pouleur H, Hanet C, Van Eyll C, Rousseau MF. Relations between global diastolic function and exercise tolerance in ischemic left ventricular dysfunction. *J Am Coll Cardiol.* 1987;9:58A.

229. Lee BH, Goodenday LS, Muswick GJ, Yasnoff WA, Leighton RF, Skell RT. Alterations of left ventricular diastolic function with doxorubicin therapy. *J Am Coll Cardiol.* 1987; 9:187-88.

230. Klein AL, Hatle LK, Burtsow DJ. Doppler characterization of left ventricular diastolic

function in cardiac amyloidosis. *J Am Coll Cardiol.* 1989;13:1017-26.

231. Fein F, Sonnenblick EH.    Diabetic   cardiomyopathy.   *Prog Cardiovasc Cis.*
1985;27:255-70.

# INDEX

# V

# W

# Y